A Case Study in Visual Agnosia Revisited

T0321021

Visual agnosia is a rare but fascinating disorder of visual object recognition that can occur after a brain lesion. This book documents the case of John, who worked intensively with the authors for 26 years after acquiring visual agnosia following a stroke. It revisits John's case over 20 years after it was originally described in the book *To See But Not To See*, in 1987. As in the previous book, the condition is illuminated by John and his wife, Iris, in their own words.

A Case Study in Visual Agnosia Revisited discusses John's case in the context of research into the cognitive neuroscience of vision over the past 20 years. It shows how John's problems in recognition can provide important insights into the way that object recognition happens in the brain, with the results obtained in studies of John's perception being compared to emerging work from brain imaging in normal observers. The book presents a much fuller analysis of the variety of perceptual problems that John experienced, detailing not only his impaired object recognition but also his face processing, his processing of different visual features (colour, motion, depth), his ability to act on and negotiate his environment, and his reading and writing.

This book will be a key reference for those concerned with understanding how vision is implemented in the brain. It will be suitable for both undergraduate students taking courses in cognitive psychology and neuropsychology, and researchers in the cognitive neuroscience of vision. The presentation of John's case, and the human aspects of the disorder, will also be of great interest to a general audience of lay people interested in perception.

Glyn Humphreys is Watts Professor of Experimental Psychology at the University of Oxford, UK. His research covers the diagnosis and management of cognitive problems after brain injury, visual attention, perception, language and the control of action, and social cognition. He has published over 500 papers in international journals and 16 books.

Jane Riddoch is Professorial Research Fellow at the University of Oxford, UK. Her research covers visual disorders (agnosia, optic aphasia), disorders of attention (neglect, extinction), and action (apraxia, action disorganisation syndrome) and neuropsychological rehabilitation. She has published 150 papers in leading international journals and authored/edited five books.

A Case Study in Visual Agnosia Revisited

To see but not to see

Second edition

Glyn Humphreys and Jane Riddoch

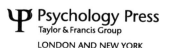

Psychology Press
Taylor & Francis Group
LONDON AND NEW YORK

Second edition published 2014
by Psychology Press
27 Church Road, Hove, East Sussex BN3 2FA

and by Psychology Press
711 Third Avenue, New York, NY 10017

Psychology Press is an imprint of the Taylor & Francis Group, an informa business

First published by Psychology Press 1987

British Library Cataloguing in Publication Data
A catalogue record for this book is available from the British Library

Library of Congress Cataloging in Publication Data
A catalog record for this book has been requested

ISBN: 978-1-84872-072-5 (hbk)
ISBN: 978-1-84872-073-2 (pbk)
ISBN: 978-0-203-55809-6 (ebk)

Typeset in Times New Roman
by Keystroke, Station Road, Codsall, Wolverhampton

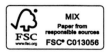

Printed and bound in Great Britain by
TJ International Ltd, Padstow, Cornwall

Contents

Figures

Plates

Preface

This book is a follow-up to an earlier book, entitled *To See But Not To See*, which we published in 1987. The original book documented the work that we had carried out up to that time with the visual agnosic patient, John. John was one of the first patients we tested when we started our research in neuropsychology. We only now realise how lucky we were to meet him. He was an amazing patient and person. As we hope will be clear through reading this book, he had a fascinating problem that disrupted his ability to recognise many objects and all faces; that destroyed his ability to see in colour and greatly disrupted his reading and his ability to find his way around. On the other hand, it left many visual processes intact, giving us a precious window into understanding distinctions between different visual operations in the brain. Not only this, but John was strikingly articulate. He was able to put into words his strange experience of 'seeing' after his brain lesion and he was able to articulate from long-term memory many of the detailed properties of objects that he could no longer access by looking at them. He was also a very dedicated servant of science. He willingly took part, with great good nature, in countless experiments over 26 and a half years – from when he suffered his stroke, through to times close to when he passed away. We learned so much from him – and not just in terms of our scientific understanding of vision.

It is interesting looking back at a book written from a cognitive neuropsychological perspective in the mid-1980s to realise how little oriented the analysis was towards the neural basis of visual recognition. In the time that has followed there has been, if not a revolution, then at least a huge increase in our understanding of how the brain processes the visual world. The role of areas such as the 'lateral occipital complex', the fusiform gyrus and the parahippocampal gyrus was poorly understand then, and while we cannot claim anything like a full understanding now, we do at least recognise their critical role. This shift in understanding is reflected in our updating of this book, where we now bring to the fore much more work looking at the neural localisation of visual function. This has certainly influenced our own views on John's problems – an example being that we no longer think of John's difficulty in finding his way as simply being another manifestation of his recognition impairment, but rather that it reflects a distinct impairment specific to the way that the brain codes visual scenes.

Along with the greater emphasis on the neural basis of visual processing, we have also tried to provide a broader coverage of our analysis of John's visual strengths and weaknesses, discussing not only object recognition but also his processing of faces, words, colour, depth, motion and his local environment. This enables us to reflect on the role of compensatory processes (e.g., the use of depth information to enhance object recognition) and on interactions that take place between different visual processes (the need for local processes to become integrated with more global object representations). The opportunity to test John over many years following his brain lesion also enabled us to analyse how visual processing can change over time, after specific perceptual operations are impaired. We started out thinking that we were looking at the static snapshot of cognitive processes bereft of critical components, but we are left with the opinion that vision is a dynamic process, constantly subject to re-calibration between perceptual processing and memory.

As was the case for the original *To See But Not To See*, our intention is that this book is of interest not just to researchers in vision, but to anyone concerned with a scientific understanding of the mind. We have thus tried to present the research carried out with John in non-technical terms and without all of the exact details of experiments – these can be found in the scientific papers in which the data have been reported (a full list is provided in the Bibliography). We also hope that the human side of the work comes across to the reader, as neuropsychology deals with people and not just 'rabbits', to use John's term. When we re-read John's definitions of objects and his statements of his difficulties, we can hear his voice and his gentle humour. We hope we are not alone in this.

Acknowledgements

On a case study that takes place over 26 and a half years, there are many people who helped and made important contributions. Drs Mary Hill and John Pattern provided the original referral to John. Recordings of John's visual fields were initially undertaken by Professor Arden from the Institute of Ophthalmology, and Chris Kennard and Trevor Crawford, both then at the London Hospital, carried out the first eye movement work. Since then, numerous colleagues have worked with us to analyse John's deficits and have contributed to the work published on John including: Nabeela Akthar, Harriet Allen, Cecille Ballaz, Jean-François Beaudoin, Muriel Boucart, Luc Boutsen, Wouter Braet, Jane Bromley, Hanna Chainay, Nick Donnelly, Martin Edwards, Daniel Fiset, Tom Freeman, Anne Giersch, Karen Lander, Rebecca Lawson, Carmel Mevorach, Katia Osswald, Cathy Price, David Punt, Philip Quinlan, Keith Ruddock, Andrew Schofield, Tom Troscianko, and Andy Young. The work covered in the book has been supported by various grants. We are particularly grateful for funding from the Stroke Association of the UK, which has provided the bedrock of our neuropsychological research since the early 1980s. The work has also been funded by several UK Research Councils, including the Biotechnical and Biological Research Council, the Economic and Social Research Council and the Medical Research Council. Support has also been given from the Human Frontiers Science Programme. The writing of the book was supported by the Leverhulme Trust.

Of course this whole programme of work would not have occurred without the great dedication and enduring enthusiasm of John and Iris. It is to their memory that this updated text is dedicated.

Chapter 1

Serendipity

If it arrives, serendipity should be grasped.

For us, serendipity happened one day in July 1981, following a lecture we had presented to some past students of Birkbeck College in London. Birkbeck is a unique institution since teaching is given only to mature students and classes are held only in the evenings. Jane had just finished her degree in Psychology at Birkbeck, having earlier trained as a physiotherapist, and she was just embarking on a PhD. Glyn was just starting out as a lecturer. We were giving a joint lecture about the work that was forming the beginnings of Jane's PhD. Arising out of her background in physiotherapy, Jane's aim was to investigate the cognitive problems that can occur in individuals who have suffered a stroke. As the PhD began, we discussed the problems in perception that stroke patients could have, which still seemed to be poorly understood. Our starting point was a study of the difficulty some patients experience in recognising objects that do not appear in their 'standard' view. The problems presented by objects in 'unusual views' was first systematically examined by Elizabeth Warrington and her colleagues [1] at the National Hospital in London just a few blocks from our base at Birkbeck. Everyone can have some problems in recognising objects in 'unusual views'. However, Warrington and Taylor showed that patients with damage to the parietal cortex, at the top and towards the back of the brain, had major problems with identifying objects in unusual views – much more than normal. We had begun to investigate why 'parietal patients' had such problems. Was this because they relied on particular aspects of objects which were obscured in the unusual views? Did the patients fail because they did not have a fall-back process, when the critical information was hidden?

In our lecture we described some of the initial experiments we were running to find out why unusual views can become difficult for parietal patients. After the lecture, a former Birkbeck graduate, Mary Hill, came up to us to describe a patient she had recently met. Mary was then working as a clinical psychologist in Guildford, and her job was to assess the many varieties of cognitive problem that can arise when the brain is damaged. In this role she had recently seen someone who seemed to have a problem in recognising all kinds of objects, not just those seen in unusual views. The interesting thing, she said, was that the patient seemed to have retained full knowledge about what objects were when he talked about them, but he was no longer able to access this knowledge when he looked at objects. He could describe what he was seeing in terms of the visual properties of the objects ('it is long and thin with a large end, and it has a shiny surface') and so he was clearly not blind. He could also describe objects from memory. However, somehow when he looked at objects, he no longer seemed able to make contact between what he was seeing and what he knew. Would we be willing to try and investigate the problem? Our moment of serendipity had arrived, though we did not know it. We said yes.

Chapter 2

Meeting in a dressing gown

Something is happening and you don't know what it is. . .

Mary Hill was kind enough to give us a referral to see John, her unusual patient. He is very nice, she said, but his wife is formidable. In the UK, the word formidable can be short-hand for a person who might be difficult. Mary informed us that we would be best advised to phone John's wife to see if she was happy for us to meet with him in order to try and clarify the problems he was having. We can still remember phoning Iris, John's wife, and wondering what we might be facing. What we found was not someone who was difficult, but rather someone who was very concerned about the problems her husband was having and wanting to understand why he had visual recognition difficulties. We told her that we were only just starting out in this area but we were very happy to come and meet her and John and to do our best to assess John's sudden visual difficulties. Iris filled us in on some of the primary symptoms – that objects could be seen well enough to be grasped, that John did not bump into things, but that he could not recognise what objects were. Once an object was grasped, however, it could be recognised. John could not identify Iris from her face, though he could identify her voice. He appeared to have lost the ability to read, and he could no longer see colours. The problem with colours was striking since John knew a lot about light and shade, as his job had involved advising museums about glass protection for their works of art.

The June day we drove down from London to Guildford was memorable in many ways – not only because we met John and Iris for the first time. To begin with, it was pouring with rain – not just English drizzle but a real hard rain bouncing off the pavement. Guildford is a town south of London with quite steep surrounding hills and John and Iris lived on one of these hills. By the time we reached the house there was a torrent of water running down the gulley at the side of the road and it was impossible to leave the car without stepping in it. Feet soaking, we then had to negotiate the steep steps that ran from the pavement down to John and Iris's house, which was some way below road height. Coming down the steps, umbrellas to the fore, Jane slipped and ended up very wet as we rang the doorbell. It was not the most professional of entrances but it certainly broke the ice!

Jane was so wet in fact that Iris made her change out of her dress and put on one of Iris's dressing gowns. The formidable lady was in fact very human! And so we began what became a constant for us and for John for the next 26 years – John sitting at a desk and we 'testing' him – giving him stimuli and assessing where his recognition succeeded and where it broke down. He, with good humour and endless patience, trying his best. We, learning.

On this first occasion, John and Iris began to explain to us what had happened. At the beginning of April John had gone into hospital for an appendix operation. After coming round from the anaesthetic, John found that he was unable to recognise the objects he was looking at, nor could he identify his son, his grandchildren or even Iris when she came in. John also found it very difficult to read the book he had brought with him and he was astonished to see that the flowers by his bedside had lost their colour. The people at the hospital at first thought that John might have been exaggerating these symptoms or that he was having some sort of nervous breakdown – in part, perhaps because the difficulties John was experiencing were so surprising after an appendix operation. He was given a brain scan using CT but this showed nothing untoward. However, as Iris insisted, John's failure to recognise things wasn't even slightly strange, it was bizarre. She was told that John's post-operative confusion would recover once he returned home, but now she was home she knew something was very wrong. The formidable side of Iris's nature would not be told 'no' and John was referred to see a clinical psychologist – Mary Hill – and following this, Mary referred him to us.

After our wet arrival, we were brought through to John and Iris's dining room and we put down on their best French-polished table the paraphernalia that then made up the tools of the trade for neuropsychologists – a large box of everyday objects, books of stimuli, even a few fruits and vegetables! We were not sure that Iris was impressed, but we started to test John in any case. One of the very rewarding things about neuropsychology is that, sometimes, it is possible to run just a few tests and to know immediately that you are faced with an amazing case. There is a striking scene in the Wes Anderson film, *The Royal Tenenbaums*, where a psychologist assesses one of the Tenenbaum children who are all supremely talented and it is immediately clear that the child is off the top of the test scale. The psychologist's face is a picture as he realises he is seeing a 'special case'. Well, those moments can occur in neuropsychology and we can all be guilty of the 'Wow, this is interesting' reaction. We were guilty here. It was clear that John could not recognise many common objects. He found our fruits and vegetables to be very difficult – he could name the banana but could not discriminate between other items that had similar shapes – whether it was a cherry, a plum or a tomato was lost to him; he confused an apple, a nectarine and an onion. This was not just a naming problem; he had difficulty deciding which of the items were fruits and which vegetables – a task that was trivial once he was given their names. He reported too that he no longer saw these stimuli in colour but only as shades of grey. The problem was not confined to fruits and vegetables; he also had difficulties in identifying pictures of other objects. However, despite not being able to identify the pictures, John was able to copy them. Figure 2.1 gives some examples of John's drawings of objects he failed to recognise. He could name some common tools but not the less familiar ones, and he could not show by gesturing how to use the implements he could not name. However, as soon as the tool was in his hands he could name it and he could demonstrate its use. John's performance was systematic and consistent – if shown the same object again, he could tell us that he'd seen that item earlier and he *still* did not know what it was! He did not bump into furniture when walking around the house and, when asked to, he reached unhesitatingly to pick up objects (as Iris tellingly remarked, even the tiniest crumbs she might have left on their carpet!).

As also noted by Iris, John had difficulty in reading. He was formerly an avid reader and crossword puzzle solver, and found his poor reading intensely frustrating. We asked him to read some sample passages from the newspaper. He could make out the letters, sometimes reading each one aloud to then name the word, but he was not able to apprehend the whole word at a glance. This process was so slow that not only John but also we, his listeners, found it was extremely difficult to remember what early parts of a passage were about, once John reached the end!

We finished our first test session by giving John a set of photographs of famous celebrities and politicians. He was unable to name any of them and said that he could only tell who was male and who female by the length of their hair or how hirsute they were – and, since the fashion at that time was for men to have long hair, even judging gender was tricky!

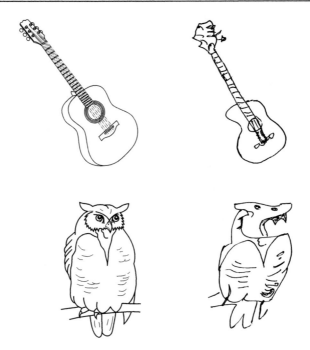

Figure 2.1 Example copies from John of stimuli he could not identify. On the left: example line drawings that John was given to identify and copy. John was unable to give any information about either the guitar or the owl and reported only that they looked like complex patterns. On the right: John's copies. The example of the owl is particularly interesting. Note that John omitted part of the owl's face on the right. In the photocopy of the drawing we gave to him, there was a small section on that part of the owl's face that was not reproduced properly. John slavishly followed that stimulus, not filling in the missing section, indicating no recognition of what the picture was.

Source: Snodgrass, J. G. and Vanderwart, M. A. (1980) cited in Humphreys, G. W. and Riddoch, M. J. (1987) *To See But Not To See: A Case of Visual Agnosia.* Hillsdale, NJ: Lawrence Erlbaum.

The problem was again not one of naming. John was putting down to chance classifying who was a politician, who was an entertainer, and so forth.

Here we were faced with an individual who could copy objects that he could neither categorise nor name from vision, who, at the same time, could name the objects when he touched them. This cluster of symptoms defines what is termed visual agnosia – 'not knowing' from vision. When this difficulty applies to faces, it is labelled 'prosopagnosia'. The apparent loss of colour perception is known as 'achromatopsia', and the loss of recognition for whole words is termed 'alexia'. These different labels reflect the fact that, although these problems can be found together, they can also sometimes occur in isolation – thus requiring separate classification labels rather than being labelled as a coherent single syndrome. In John's case, however, it was apparent that he had all of these problems – and there were other difficulties we were yet to discover, such as not being able to find his way around both familiar and unfamiliar environments (so-called 'topographical agnosia'). We were able to explain to John and Iris that these strange symptoms were known to sometimes co-occur and that they almost certainly were the result of the stroke that John had suffered. He had had a devastating thing happen to him, but he wasn't undergoing a breakdown. Sometimes having a problem identified and labelled can be a reassurance – even if the label doesn't really explain why faces and words were strikingly difficult or why John could apparently see objects well enough to draw them but still failed to recognise what they were. Our aim was to try and provide some answers as to why these problems arose. For John and Iris, the initial aim was to take on board what had happened, which they did admirably. We asked if we could return to try and explore John's problems in greater detail. They agreed. Later they were kind enough to say they would have agreed even if they had known the years of further tests that would subsequently be undertaken.

Chapter 3

On becoming agnosic

The day I arrived with flowers and he asked what they were.

(Iris)

Until April 1981, the course of John's life was not dissimilar from that of many other lives. It had had its high spots and low spots, its moments of personal happiness and success, its moments of failure. John was educated at a boarding school in England while his parents were abroad in India. He came of age just as the Second World War was starting and he trained to be an aeroplane pilot. He spent the initial part of the Second World War stationed in France with the RAF, and was later involved as a fighter pilot during the Battle of Britain. Subsequently he transferred to the army and became a member of the tank regiment, going over to Germany after the Normandy invasion. One of his favourite stories was of when he directed a tank across the thin struts of a temporary bridge crossing the Rhine – after which he celebrated with a bottle of champagne! During the war he married Iris. Following the war, he worked in a firm engaged in the manufacture of metal windows for houses. He was later employed by an American company which was concerned with the control of solar heat and ultra-violet radiation. He rose to an executive position, and had responsibility for marketing within Europe. He knew a lot about light and colour.

In 1981, John's life changed dramatically after he had been taken in for an emergency appendix operation. Post-operatively, he suffered a stroke – a conclusion later confirmed through MRI analyses, but this was not known at the time, and indeed an initial CT scan had failed to show any problem. Unfortunately, CT scans can sometimes miss a lesion if they are performed too early after a stroke, and that was the case for John. John had had a history of atrial fibrillation (uneven contractions of the upper chambers of the heart). It is possible that this heart condition could have resulted in a small blood clot travelling to the brain, blocking one of the arteries supplying the brain and causing the death of brain tissue. Stroke is perhaps most commonly associated with paralysis on one side of the body (termed a hemiplegia) or with a problem in speech (aphasia). In John's case, the damage was in the region of the posterior cerebral artery, affecting the occipital lobes at the back of the brain (see Figure 3.1 on p. 15, for an MRI scan of John's brain, taken in 2005). Since the occipital lobes are quite removed from the regions controlling movement and speech, damage there does not produce the associated paralysis or speech problems which are more commonly found after stroke. John had no difficulties in walking or in moving his arms and hands; he was able to understand conversations and he was articulate in describing the problems he was experiencing. Given that there were not the usual signs of stroke, and that a stroke was unexpected after an appendectomy, the cause of his problem was not immediately detected. From the point of view of the medical personnel, John did behave in a very odd way. He did not recognise the doctors and nurses who attended him, he would get lost when trying to find his way to the bathroom even though he had been shown the way several times, and he complained that he was unable to read. There is always some degree of stress associated with surgery, and it is not unknown for patients subsequently to show a degree of confusion and disorientation. These symptoms, however, usually do not persist, and medical staff are trained to provide reassurance for as long as the symptoms last. John was given such reassurance, but unfortunately his confusion did not abate. John's recollection of the early days painted a clear picture. He wrote:

> My first memory is being aware of that dreadful unending clatter of clashing metal containers, cutlery and serving trolleys, ringing in apparently hypersensitive ears, mingling with that sickening, all-pervading smell of cheap 'general' disinfectant which told my slowly awakening brain that I was in a hospital. Of that I was categorically certain; the sounds and smells were instantly acceptable. I don't suppose the events of the next few minutes were much different to the normal return to full consciousness after any anaesthesia. The most puzzling next event was my wife's first visit. I recognised her voice quite easily, but put down to some sort of hangover any certainty of seeing her properly. On her leaving, I remember quite clearly assuring myself that some temporary 'bang on the head' was affecting my vision.

Because I was in hospital, I was presented at breakfast time with a menu showing what was on offer for the next two days and I was asked to mark my ticket for the next half-dozen meals. Because I was kept very well changed and shaven, etc. by my visiting wife, it was assumed by the nurses that I must be a difficult patient because I kept handing back the menu cards uncompleted. It was my wife who discovered that I had completely lost the ability to read. Thank goodness, though, she had the sense and determination to return the very next day with a pack of 'lexicon' cards. She literally started by having me read single letters and then two- or three-letter words.

When something totally inexplicable happens, the overriding initial response is to hope it will go away while continuing with everyday activities in as normal a fashion as possible. It is reasonable to think then that, because John was trying to cope with each new problem as it arose, he was unable to appreciate the overall magnitude of the situation. The same was not true of Iris who quickly became painfully aware of the totality of the difficulties John was experiencing. Her dismay was clearly expressed:

A day or two after my husband's operation I knew something was seriously wrong. The medical and nursing staff assured me that he was just suffering from post-operative shock, but this did not allay my fears. Each day when I visited him, there was additional evidence of his problems. The fact that he would ask visitors, at short intervals, what the time or day was, and could not remember what he had eaten for lunch a few minutes previously was strange, but I thought this could be post-operative shock. However, the day I arrived with flowers and he asked what they were really worried me, and caused me to ask what colour they and the curtains of the ward were. Grey was the reply, and a few further questions ascertained that suddenly he was completely colour-blind.

That night I went home distressed, knowing that I had to face the fact that, whatever the doctors said, something had affected his brain and life for him would never be the same again. I knew he had not been able to see the sketches or read the words on his get-well cards, and I spent the night thinking of ways in which I could help him. Next day I took in some 'lexicon' cards and when I asked him the names of the letters, he got several wrong. Each day I continued this game and gradually he could read words of three letters. He would spell them out letter by letter: 'm', 'a', 'p', 'map' – though sometimes this would become 'mad' not 'map'. Longer words at this stage defeated him.

Encouraged by the fact that he could remember events months or years before, I gave him a piece of paper and asked him to sign his name. Imagine my joy and relief when he produced a perfect signature quickly and with all the usual dots and loops! I followed this up by suggesting that he wrote a few lines to thank someone for their good wishes. This was not a good effort, some words were repeated, and some letters such as 'p' and 'd' or 's' or 'z' were mixed up. He was also unable to read back what he had written, so, after an interruption for a cup of tea, I had to read back the last sentence. Unfortunately an hour afterwards he had forgotten he had written it and asked me to write to his friend.

He had been moved to a ward with only six or eight beds, but was upset because he could not find his way to the cloakroom. At Easter, other patients in the ward were allowed home for the holiday so for two hours we were able to walk backwards and forwards to the cloakroom to try to learn the route. In the end he was able to manage the trip by himself, so next day I asked his ward mate whether he had gone there by himself.

'No, he had to be brought back from the corridor', was the disappointing reply.

The neurologists were troubled by his lack of progress and thought that a return to his home surroundings would be helpful, so four weeks after the operation, arrangements were made for his wound to be dressed at home and he was discharged.

Being unsure of his reactions to a car journey, I asked a friend to drive us in his car and kept John talking to keep his mind off the traffic.

'Why do we stop here?' he asked when the car stopped.

'You live here,' I replied.

'Really?' he answered.

We walked into the house and he looked around as though he had never been there before. After some days he could find his way from room to room but could not recognise ornaments, pictures or furniture. It seemed important to him to feel he could do some things unaided so for several days I took him to the post box, about 50 yards down the road on the same side of the street. One day I suggested he could save me time by going to the post on his own. Watching from the window I saw him walk quite confidently in the right direction and all went well until on the return trip, he walked past the house. Luckily we lived at the end of a cul-de-sac so he realised his error and turned back but stood for many minutes at the top of our steps before deciding that it was our house.

John's return home, for him, led to a realisation that he had a significant problem in recognising people, objects, and his everyday environment. He described it thus:

I have to say that my first few days back at home caused such a disappointment with the firmly expressed medical opinion that 'all would click back quite simply', that in some ways confidence in anyone became more restricted. This period lasted some time, during which I fell into tantrums caused by very minor problems following my inability to carry out simple everyday tasks, and most particularly if I read criticism into a comment or action. One of our few remaining pleasures at the time was minding the dogs of a friend. Whilst doing this one weekend I read criticism into some very innocent comment from my wife and just swept the whole kitchen tableload of china to the floor, and flounced off into the garden like some hysterical girl – behaviour unlikely and most certainly disproved by my grandfather status. During my first few months at home, various such flare-ups occurred; they were short-lasting. On one occasion I lost my temper whilst helping my wife in the garden. Again I read 'complaint' into something she said. By mischance, I had a long-handled garden fork in my hands, and promptly threw it – well, perhaps if not directly at her, then very near her, where it stuck into the ground. I stormed off out of the garden, onto the nearby common hillside, and stamped across to the woodlands edging it. I reached there in perhaps a few minutes, breathless, and was then rapidly 'cooled off' by the realisation that I had no idea how to get home again; it was no good looking back; I knew there was a gate into the grassed area from the road where the house stood, but I could not recognise it. My hot temper cooled very rapidly as I had to work out from memory that as long as I travelled downhill and followed the line of the trees and undergrowth that bordered three sides of the grassy hillside, I could reach the wicket gate into our road. Fortunately though, I didn't have to make the journey alone as my better half had already set off to rescue me! I cite these as a couple of the more ludicrous actions I took during the initial few months after returning home.

John had been discharged home in the hope that familiar surroundings might decrease his post-operative 'confusion'. His symptoms continued, though. He was unable to recognise familiar faces, the familiar objects around his home were misidentified, he got lost when he ventured outside. He could only read slowly and with great effort, and, though he could write, he often could not read back what he had written; he had also lost the ability to see colour. The world became black and white and shades of grey.

Iris found it hard to believe that some neurological incident had not occurred in view of John's strikingly abnormal behaviour. She wrote to John's doctor:

I find it hard to accept that John's visual difficulties could be accounted for by a nervous breakdown but then my knowledge of such things is nil! He is still totally colour-blind and he cannot tell the difference between different leaf shapes or differentiate between flowers and leaves in the garden which prevents him enjoying his favourite hobby of gardening. He still cannot recognise even me by sight and if waiting for me outside a shop will look blankly or perhaps uncertainly at me until I speak. He does not see pictures and cannot describe the subject matter of those we have had in the house for years. His reading is restricted to newspaper headlines or larger print books which he can tolerate for only short periods before his eyes start watering. The speed of reading is very slow. As reading was another favourite relaxation, he finds this disability very frustrating.

His letter writing has improved. The first attempts contained a number of repeated words but this now seldom happens. He does, however, sometimes write the wrong letters, the most frequent being 'p' for 'd' or 'z' for 's' and he often mixes up 'p' for 'd' when he reads aloud to me.

His factual long-term memory seems reasonable and he can converse well. We do the D.T.[1] crossword puzzles with me reading the clues; he contributes quite a good number of answers, remembering books, quotations and odd words. He can also recall the names of men and facts about jobs connected with his past business. Contrary to this, he cannot find his way around Guildford or recognise any roads when we drive around the local area which he has known for over 20 years. After about four trips I now let him go to the post box 30 yards away on the same side of the street as at last he has learnt to recognise our house. Sometimes in the town he thinks he knows where he is but unfortunately he is more likely to be wrong than right.

The short-term memory is still giving him problems but more so when associated with sight. He is continually putting things in the wrong place even if I tell him where they go a minute before. If I ask him to fetch a glass or cup, he opens nearly every cupboard in the kitchen before finding the right one. To solve the problem of him not remembering how to turn the TV or radio on, I had to put white adhesive tape on the 'on' button. He can see the TV but describes it as a poor black and white picture and does not recognise the faces . . .

Thanks to Iris's persistence and the subsequent referrals that were made, more detailed tests of John's condition were carried out. Subsequent CT and MRI scans carried out in 1982 and then again in 1985 and 2005 were able to confirm that a stroke had taken place. An MRI scan of John's brain is shown in Figure 3.1 which indicates that John had suffered lesions on both sides to the back, lower regions of the brain. In Chapter 4 we will describe how the regions affected are precisely those that support our visual recognition of the world. Given the location of the damage, it is not surprising that John suffered major problems in recognition when he came round after his operation – the problem was physiological, not psychological. Tests of John's basic vision demonstrated that he had normal acuity on standard letter charts but that he was blind in some areas of his visual field. In particular, John could not detect stimuli presented above the central meridian in either eye. The fact that there was a field loss in both eyes is telling, and it points to him having a central brain lesion rather than the damage being more peripheral, for instance, affecting just one of his eyes or the optic nerves. Vision from the two eyes only becomes integrated within the brain, so that damage to the brain can lead to problems in seeing in both eyes. The loss of vision in his upper visual fields arose because his lesions were to lower brain regions (the upper parts of the retina projects to these brain areas). However, this visual field loss, alone, is not sufficient to explain John's difficulties in recognition. It does mean that when he looked at someone's eyes, he may not have seen the top of their head; likewise when he looked at the door of a house, he would not see the roof.

On the other hand, John had no difficulty in making eye movements or head movements, and with slight adjustments, all of the visual field could fall into his intact areas of vision. Indeed, John's excellent ability to copy objects, illustrated in the previous chapter (see Figure 2.1),

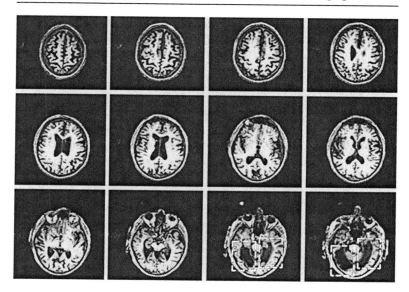

Figure 3.1 An MRI scan of John's brain. The front of the brain is shown at the top and the back of the brain at the bottom of each horizontal slice. The slices start at the top of the brain and are then taken at progressively lower cuts. John's nose and eyes are visible at the top of the slices in the lowest row. The brain lesions are indicated by the white rectangles drawn on the scans. There are lesions on both sides of the brain (bilateral lesions), and they occur at relatively low regions within what is known as the 'ventral' (lower) cortex. As we shall discuss in Chapter 4, the lesions affect brain areas involved in the visual processing of objects, faces, colour and places.

indicates that the problem was not one of blindness or not seeing; rather, there was a problem in interpreting information after it had been detected. This difficulty in interpreting the visual world is illustrated by an example of John's behaviour noted by one of the doctors: 'Whilst weeding, he will disturb his wife by pulling out the annual planting, yet he will cut a hedge without difficulty – but then he will continue with the shears straight into the roses.' In some senses, John could 'see' – he was able to cut a hedge without difficulty – but he had problems in visual *recognition* – he failed to discriminate plants from weeds, or the hedge from the rose bushes.

Establishing that some sort of damage exists is, however, is only the beginning of the story. We need to know exactly what processes in vision have become difficult, if we are to explain what is going wrong and if we are to draw lessons from John's case about how recognition operates. To give some insights into the problems of everyday life in agnosia, we asked John to answer a set of verbal questions about his experience. As we hope to show when we describe our more formal analyses of John's recognition (see Chapter 6), some of John's insights into his problems were uncannily correct and give beautiful illustrations of the types of visual processing impairment present in agnosic patients.

Are you able to describe your visual problem to us?

To try and explain how I see the world is quite difficult; somehow what I am seeing can't be easily captured in words. If I try hard, the nearest description I can get to is to say that everything is slightly out of focus, though not to my eyes if you understand, but to my brain. However, this is really inadequate. I know from an optical point of view that my lens-corrected vision is as good as can be achieved – my vision has been extensively examined to ensure that there were no obvious reasons which might inhibit my recognition of things. I therefore harbour no irrational ideas that there will be any sudden cure, such as the design of some new glasses.

How do you manage with the recognition of common objects?

I have come to cope with recognising many common objects, if they are standing alone, and I manage by trying to keep things in the same place – just as if I were blind. When objects are placed together, though, I have more difficulties. For instance, eating at a buffet or self-service restaurant is extremely difficult, especially bearing in mind that I only see in black and white. One time, at a buffet, I mistook horse-radish sauce for cream and poured it on my strawberries – only to be unpleasantly surprised! Also, although I can recognise many food items seen individually, they somehow seem hard to separate en masse. To recognise one sausage on its own is far from picking one out from a dish of cold foods in a salad: a case of can't see the trees for the wood?

Are some cues easier than others?

Generally, I find moving objects much easier to recognise than static images, presumably because I see different and changing views – it is a normal human reaction, after all, to give oneself several different and moving views of an unknown object when trying to recognise it. For that reason the TV screen enables me to comprehend far more of an outdoor scene than, for example, the drawings on my living room walls which I have known for a lifetime, but now cannot recognise.

For many years an excellent etching of St Paul's Cathedral in London has hung on our living room wall – drawn by an outstanding member of the Academy of Royal Arts – depicting the bomb-cleared era of London during the 39–45 war [see Figure 3.2]. I know the building has the famous dome-shaped roof and I can point it out in detail on the picture. But now it does not 'fit' my memory of the picture nor of the reality. With my knowledge of the building, I should be able to identify it from its general design. There should be a dome-headed, high central circular tower covering a cruciform layout. I can see this in my mind. And, when I look at the etching, I can point out the expected detail but I cannot recognise the whole structure. On the other hand, I am sure I could draw a reasonable copy of the picture. The reason I say this is that I can see very clearly every detail of the objects even if I do not always recognise the whole. Pictures are much more difficult if the artist has used shade, reflection or the skills of Impressionism (rather than directly portraying trees, water or a cloudscape, say).

Mostly, I am able to recognise the general class that an object belongs to – such as whether it is an animal or a bird; but I cannot tell which particular animal or bird it is. The problem is not confined to animate objects. For instance, we recently went to the RAF museum at Hendon. I knew well in advance I was to see an old

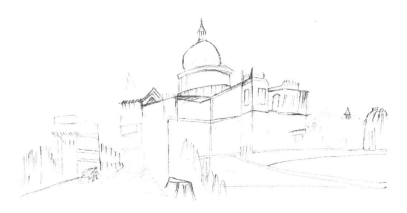

Figure 3.2 John's copy of an etching of St Paul's Cathedral in London during the Blitz, which he refers to in his description above

Source: From Humphreys, G. W. and Riddoch, M. J. (1987) *To See But Not To See: A Case of Visual Agnosia.* Hillsdale, NJ: Lawrence Erlbaum.

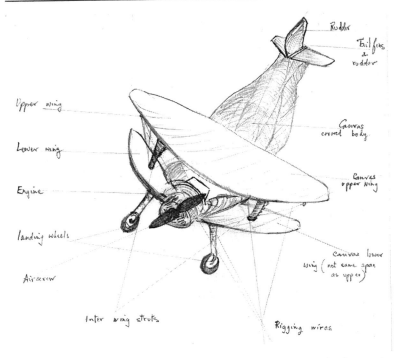

Figure 3.3 John's drawing from memory of a Lysander plane which he flew at the start of the Second World War

Source: From Humphreys, G. W. and Riddoch, M. J. (1987) *To See But Not To See: A Case of Visual Agnosia*. Hillsdale, NJ: Lawrence Erlbaum.

Lysander which I used to fly in '39–40 (until I went into the army). Now, a Lysander is very different in general shape from most aircraft ever made and distinguishable to a degree [see Figure 3.3]. The odd thing was that when we came to the display, I did not see it 'in toto'. I recalled enough to tell the others to pick out details and where to find them and had them laughing when I remembered the ludicrous instructions for the rear gunner to bale out in a hurry, etc., and even where certain equipment not on display used to be fitted. Still I did not recognise the 'whole'.

Although you are not able to recognise objects when you see them, are you able to remember what a particular object should look like?

To draw from memory I don't find too difficult, bearing in mind that I never had much drawing ability or the simplest comprehension of how to show a third dimension in scribbling.[2] On the other hand, my mind knows very clearly what I should like to draw and I can comprehend enough of my own handiwork to know if it is a reasonable representation of what I had in mind. However, there are a few objects I cannot recall to mind – particularly some flowers, for which I remember the botanical names but not their appearance.

What about recognising faces?

Probably my most embarrassing problem is not recognising people. Since coming round I have never been able to recognise any person by sight alone. I cannot recognise my wife except by the sound of her voice, nor my grandchildren, nor my family nor friends. I also have great problems with animals, particularly if they are not moving.

Friends and business acquaintances of long standing, like the milkman and the GP, I can recognise by sound. Of my generation, most of the men wear their trousers of instep length and sport haircuts shorter than their wives and daughters. I frequently free the inner side of pavements to long-haired, short-trousered boys who probably have no conception of convention anyway!

I have learned that to recognise people it's often easiest to use non-facial clues – an obvious example is hair length and general pattern. My problem in seeing colour can also cause extra difficulties as I don't differentiate between blondes and grey-haired ladies. I recall mannerisms shown by friends and family – the use of arms when speaking, ear scratching, ways of standing, all visual aids to identify them in parties and groups where auditory clues are too confused or numerous for separation.

Awaiting my wife's exit from supermarkets, I have astonished strange ladies by picking up their shopping and walking away with it, under the impression that it was my wife I had been watching pass through the pay desk! On occasion, when travelling to town, she or my grandchildren ask me to identify animals in the fields: if the animals are static, I'm often wrong. The same goes for buildings. Even with major London buildings I'm often at a loss except for very obvious and clear standing examples like the Albert Hall, which I can get from its dome.

Are you able to recognise yourself in a mirror?

Well, I can certainly see a face, with eyes, nose and mouth, etc., but somehow it's not familiar; it really could be anybody. I can also see enough to decide whether my now-limited hair is tidy or in need of a brush, but at the same time as this I don't seem to have enough detail to know whether I need a shave or whether my face is dirty. But I can see the tiny scarred notch on my nose and recall how and where it was caused, years ago.

What about colour vision?

I only see objects in shades of grey. This lack of colour vision is quite annoying in relationship to everyday living. I am unsure of matching pairs of socks of similar length and fabric, and certainly I am bad at choosing the appropriate tie for a shirt or jacket.

Are you able to read?

Of all my problems, I find that, being reduced to reading so slowly, the most frustrating on an everyday basis. The problem simplified is that the mental exercise in making sense of the letters in order to create a word requires so much effort that I have often forgotten the overall content of a sentence by the time I get to the end, requiring re-reading in order to comprehend the whole. I also find great difficulty in reading my own longhand, let alone that of others.

How do you manage to find your way about?

This is another major problem. An extension of my initial problem of not knowing the geography of my house is a still continuing difficulty of not recognising my surroundings and consequently not knowing my whereabouts. A small collection of shops is about 240 paces away from the entrance of the flat we have moved to.[3] I know this because it took my patient wife more than 12 months teaching before I could do it 'solo'. The post office is about 10 minutes' walk away; I am now convinced that I could find my way there, but my instructor will not yet trust me! Along with this there is a subsidiary difficulty. I am not good at judging distances or the speed of road traffic, so we tend to be cautious in sending me out for errands! Also, because of this problem with distances and speeds, I am an incredibly bad front seat passenger. The generality of my discomfort in this situation arises from my own conviction that the car is much nearer to the vehicle in front than is really true. When I go to the shops I can manage perfectly well until I meet friends en route and stop to chat. I can then be quite disoriented, and I have to reorient myself either by asking them or walking on until I recognise a salient point from which to continue the journey. Quite recently, due to 'not thinking what I was doing', I had to return to my last recognised checkpoint, our block of flats, to recommence the short journey to the shops.

It has crossed family minds as to what I should do were I to get badly lost in a town, during normal hours, I would just ask a passer-by, take a taxi home, or if I were really desperate, find my way by asking a policeman! I have not yet had to do this, but I hope I could explain my predicament to the puzzled public! Fortunately, I have not lost my social skills and I could find a hotel in a strange town and am quite capable of organising an overnight room and meals until I could be rescued. I have also not become fearful in public places but rather hypercritical of the ill manners – imagined or otherwise – of people. I suppose I have turned out to be rather crustier than I should, but that has always been the privilege of seniority.

Starting from here

John's descriptions provide striking examples of what it is like to be agnosic. His introspections indicate something of the strangeness and the frustration of being deserted by the normally automatic processes of visual recognition. It describes a visual world full of pitfalls and booby traps – where the eye and attention are guided to parts of an image that do not convey the key information present. It describes a constant state of being led down the visual garden path, so to speak. From this starting place we may try to unpick the processes that are going wrong, to help us understand how these processes might normally operate and what role they play in our everyday visual encounters. In this visual journey we were indeed lucky to work with John. From the early days immediately after his stroke until his death in 2008, we saw John from between three to six times a year. He and Iris became close friends of our family as is indicated by the closing paragraph of a letter he wrote to us in September 1991 in which he sent good wishes to our children: 'My respectful greetings to Miss the Junior monitor and encouraging growls to the hardworking (?) boys . . .'. While we lived in London, we used to travel down to Guildford for a day of testing with John. We were always warmly greeted by Iris with freshly made coffee and homemade biscuits. Testing was carefully structured with the most demanding tasks being administered before lunch as John always delighted in his pre-lunch sherry, and enjoyed a glass of wine with his meal. The lunches were always delicious. Iris was an expert on home economics, and she went to great lengths in her preparations – we have never tasted a better steak and kidney pie! On occasion, when specialist equipment was necessary for our tests, John and Iris would travel up to London and they delighted to tell friends about the time we stopped to have a picnic on Waterloo Bridge. They said this was done solely because we would not waste the lunch break but rather could continue asking John to identify the buildings that could be seen from this vantage point – a claim that was not entirely true! Later we moved to new positions at the University of Birmingham and John and Iris came up to stay with us – with John going through full days of testing before gaining his well-earned glass of wine at the end! As any of our colleagues who had the pleasure of working with John would attest, he was a terrific 'observer' – very consistent in his judgements and serious in his performance (would that undergraduates were always as dedicated!). But lest it sound as if we made unreasonable impositions on him, John was later to write:

> I have welcomed being a research rabbit for some time. I have been so surprised at the broad spread of experiments and exercises to which I have been subject. Over the years I have seen the incredible advances in the tools and impedimenta used to test and time reactions to visual stimuli, but it remains a layman's delight to me to note how frequently a session will end with pencilled graphs and diagrams on the back of old envelopes. To myself, the unqualified onlooker, ripples in a still pond perhaps!

John and Iris's attitude made research a particular pleasure.

Notes

1 *The Daily Telegraph* is a British daily newspaper.
2 Despite John's modesty, his copying and drawing from memory do suggest considerable artistic talent!
3 It is interesting that John describes this distance in terms of paces, presumably reflecting his fall-back strategy for finding his way around.

Chapter 4

The visual brain

Lights flicker from the opposite loft. . .

To begin to understand the problems experienced by John, we need to introduce some of the research from cognitive neuroscience that has informed views of how the brain recognises the visual world.

The fragmentation of vision

The brain is comprised of grey matter, the neurons that become active when we sense, think and act, and white matter, within which the fibre tracts are housed that conduct activity between neurons in different parts of the brain. There is also grey matter found in evolutionarily-old 'sub-cortical' structures found underneath the cerebral cortex, which forms the multi-folded surface of the brain (Figure 4.1). The cortex is the seat of our main 'higher order' cognitive functions – speaking and understanding, solving problems, recognising objects and people. It is conventionally divided into four main 'lobes', each replicated in each cerebral hemisphere: the occipital lobes at the back, the parietal lobes which go forward from the occipital lobes towards the top of the brain, the temporal lobes at the side of the brain, and the frontal lobes, which form the anterior (front) parts of the cortex. The occipital lobes receive sensory information from the eyes and are the starting point for our analysis of the visual brain.

Much of our early knowledge about the neural basis of visual processing came from animal studies where recordings were made from single neurons firing in response to visual input or where investigators examined the effects of selective brain lesions. Pioneering single cell recording studies were carried out by the subsequent Nobel Prize-winners, David

Figure 4.1 The left hemisphere of the human brain. The back of the brain is on the right and the front on the left.

Source: From Eysenck, M. E. (2013) *Simply Psychology*, 3rd edn. Hove: Psychology Press, p. 42. reprinted by permission of the publisher (Taylor & Francis Group, http://www.informaworld.com).

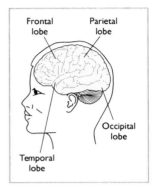

Hubel and Torsten Wiesel [2], who recorded from neurons in the primary visual cortex in the occipital lobe – the initial site in the cortex where activity on the retina is projected to. Hubel and Wiesel reported that neurons in this brain region respond selectively to edges at different orientations and to different spatial frequencies (crudely, widths) of patterns. Thus one cell might respond strongly to a vertical edge but not to a horizontal edge, while another might show the opposite response profile. The cells were also found to be arranged in a systematic fashion, providing a 'retinotopic map' of the world. In this map, neighbouring neurons respond to stimuli at neighbouring locations on the retina. The fact that the primary visual cortex codes a retinal map reflecting spatial layout in the world can explain why individuals can become blind to stimuli in one part of space after damaging their visual cortex – essentially that part of their retinotopic map is no longer registered by the brain, so that information from that region is not fed forward to other brain regions involved in object recognition. This represents a form of cortical blindness. It was due to damage to such a retinotopic map in his brain that John could no longer see in his upper parts of his visual fields. Since Hubel and Wiesel's pioneering work, over 30 different visually responsive areas have been documented, defined by different physical properties (e.g., the histology of the cells), by the cells showing contrasting response preferences to different stimuli and (in some cases) the re-duplication of a retinotopic map (with several areas each coding their own separate map) [3].

Within some of these regions the cells show quite selective responses – they may respond to one but not another colour and to some but not other directions of motion [4]. For example, in the brain region V4, which falls along a lower pathway (often termed the ventral pathway) from the occipital lobe to the temporal lobe, neurons have a selective response to colour but show minimal selectivity to motion – they may respond to red but not green, but do not care whether the stimulus moves or is static. This can be contrasted with the responses of cells in area MT, which falls within a pathway higher up the brain, from occipital cortex into posterior parietal cortex (typically termed the *dorsal* visual pathway). Cells in area MT have motion selectivity but minimal colour selectivity – they may fire if a stimuli moves in one but not another direction, but they are insensitive to whether the stimulus is red or green [4]. Cells in the posterior parietal cortex also respond selectively to stimuli at different binocular depths and in relation to specific actions that might be prepared to a stimulus, suggesting that this brain region is critically involved in using visual information for reaching in depth and for visually-guided action [5]. These results suggest that, at a cortical level, the brain parcels up visual stimuli so that there is specialised processing of contrasting features (such as colour, depth and motion) in different brain regions. Furthermore the information coded in different regions may also be used for contrasting purposes, for example, to recognise an object or to establish where it is in space. One classic distinction, introduced by Ungerleider and Mishkin [6], is between the brain areas involved in coding 'what' a stimulus is (areas in the ventral pathway, from the occipital cortex into the temporal lobe) and 'where' a stimulus is (areas in the dorsal pathway from the occipital to the parietal lobe). Ungerleider and Mishkin's conclusions came from studies looking at the effects of selectively lesioning the ventral and dorsal pathways in monkeys (Figure 4.2, Plate 1 in the plate section). Damage to the ventral pathway disrupts the ability of a monkey to discriminate between different objects but they can remember *where* to go to in order to obtain a reward. In contrast, lesioning the dorsal pathway impairs associations to a location, but not to *which* object was presented. Remarkably, although our visual awareness is of a coherent world of linked objects, colours and movement, with different objects seen at particular locations, processing within the brain is very different. In the brain, different features (colours, movement, objects, spatial position) are coded in distinct neural regions!

The single cell recording work conducted in non-human animals has been extended by studies using functional brain imaging of humans. Functional brain imaging measures activity in the brain while people are carrying out different tasks, with the aim being to identify the areas that are involved in the tasks. The early work on human brain imaging relied on Positron Emission Tomography (PET), where scans detect the strength of a brief-lasting radioactive oxygen isotope which is injected into the bloodstream and taken up into brain. Active brain areas use more oxygen and hence measures of the oxygen present in different brain areas index how active those regions are in tasks. More recently studies have been undertaken using functional magnetic resonance imaging (fMRI) which is non-invasive (using magnetic fields rather than X-rays), and which generates higher-resolution images over a shorter time period than PET, see [7]. Studies using PET and fMRI have largely confirmed that the processing of different visual features is distributed across a variety of brain areas. For example, Zeki and colleagues used PET to isolate colour and motion-selective responses in the human brain [8]. Participants viewed either a set of coloured squares (like a painting by the Belgian artist Mondrian) or a grey-level version of the same image, matched for brightness. The brain activity when observers viewed the grey-level image was subtracted from the activity when the coloured Mondrians were viewed, to reveal the regions that were selectively activated by the presence of colour (showing significantly greater activation for the coloured Mondrian over its grey-level baseline). The results are shown in Figure 4.3 (Plate 2 in the plate section). There was a region within the ventral visual pathway that was selectively activated by the coloured stimulus. This is the colour-responsive region V4 in humans.

Zeki and colleagues also included a further condition in their PET study in which they contrasted brain activity when observers looked at moving sets of random dots compared with when the same dots were stationary. The brain areas more active for the moving relative to the stationary displays are depicted in Figure 4.4 (see Plate 3 in the plate section). In this case, subtracting the activity associated with stationary dots from that found when the dots were moving, revealed regions in a lateral part of the occipital cortex in both hemispheres – the human area MT, where the neurons respond to motion more than to stationary stimuli.

While single cell recording studies have taught us a great deal about the processing of basic visual features (edge orientations, colours, motion), information about the further stages of visual processing (such as how these features are integrated, or about the neural steps involved in going from the coding of basic visual features to the recognition of whole objects) as yet is not as clearly specified. A problem here is that any given visually-driven cell, especially in the early cortical regions (V1, V2, V3, etc.) may only respond to stimuli falling in a small region on the retina, making it difficult to judge how multitudes of cells work together when complex stimuli such as objects and faces are recognised. For example, given that there may be many thousands of edges present in an image,

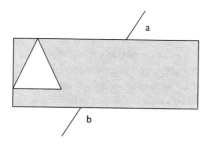

Figure 4.5 A simple example to illustrate the principles which govern inter-actions between the brain regions responding to different parts of a visual image

how does the brain know which of the features go together to make up one object and not another? What if the edges cross, as when one object is partially hidden behind another – how does the brain know which edge should go with which? Consider Figure 4.5. Why is it that we tend to see the physically separate diagonal lines as belonging together and being occluded by (rather than connecting with) the edges making up the grey rectangle? Why do we spontaneously interpret the small grey triangle in the top left of the larger rectangle as belonging to the rectangle and not as a separate shape – yet we interpret the larger white triangle as a separate shape on the left side of the rectangle?

From parts to wholes

The question of how different features in an image are combined to enable object recognition to take place was one that much concerned the Gestalt psychologists, working in the early twentieth century. These psychologists argued that object recognition was based on 'rules' that determined how local features combined into the 'perceptual units' that we see (the separate diagonal lines on either side of the rectangle in Figure 4.5 being coded as a single 'unit' – an occluded diagonal line). The 'Gestalt principles' state that elements are organised into perceptual units based on factors such as proximity (proximal elements tend to be assigned to the same perceptual unit), similarity (elements that have similar properties – e.g., elements on the grey surface of the rectangle in Figure 4.5 – will tend to be coded as belonging together), and collinearity (edges that that are aligned in the image will be coded as part of the same unit, even if physically separated – the diagonal line in Figure 4.5 being an example). These principles can be thought of as a set of 'rules' that constrain how local visual elements are combined to form the objects that we act upon in the world. The rules themselves may be embodied in the interactions between neurons based on the brain learning the 'non-accidental' statistics of the environment, i.e., the patterns of variation in the image that reflect regularities in the world. Hebbian learning [9] is a simple form of learning that could be critical. Named after the Canadian psychologist Donald Hebb who originally proposed the principle, Hebbian learning involves strengthening the connections between neurons if the neurons fire together. If a strong connection is formed between two neurons, then activation of one neuron will tend to drive the other into an active state, making the brain 'resonate' to stimuli that occur regularly in the world. This idea can be used to explain Gestalt principles such as 'similarity'. Local patches on the surfaces of objects will tend to have similar properties, for example, they will be the same colour or they will have the same texture (Figure 4.6). Neighbouring neurons that represent the same colour or texture are thus likely to fire together when an object's surface is present, increasing their connectivity. In contrast to this, when objects are not present, then neighbouring parts of an image

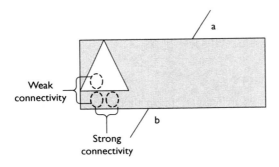

Figure 4.6 An illustration of the hypothetical neural response to similar elements at neighbouring locations. The dashed circles illustrate regions of the visual field linked to neighbouring visual neurons in the brain. Neurons responding to similar features at nearby locations will tend to be activated together when objects are present, leading to increased connectivity. Dissimilar features, being less likely to co-occur, will not co-activate neighbouring neurons so regularly, so neighbouring neurons responding to these features (white and grey regions in the figure) will have weaker connections and so are less likely to fire together. Co-activity between neurons can be used to assign visual regions to the same perceptual unit.

may be unrelated, and so neurons responding to these properties will tend not to fire together. The consequence of this is that neurons will respond most strongly together to parts of images that co-occur in objects. Hence the brain may learn to organise elements into the perceptual units that form objects.

It has also been noted that as one progresses from the primary visual areas in the occipital cortex to more anterior regions in the temporal lobe (Figures 4.1 and 4.2), so the neurons tend to have larger 'receptive fields' – meaning that the neurons no longer respond only when the appropriate feature is in a particular retinal location, but also when the feature falls across a variety of locations. The neurons in these 'higher order' areas also respond to more complex groups of features than those in primary visual cortex [10]. The responses of cells in these higher-order regions of the temporal lobe can be accounted for if the neurons pool together activity coming from many cells in the lower-level regions. The lower-level neurons respond to simple features in specific locations; the higher-order neurons combine this incoming activity to respond to more complex properties in a manner that is 'position invariant'. We can picture this as a hierarchy of processes, going from the coding of the local elements to the coding of whole objects. We term this *a parts-based approach* to object processing, in which the brain responds to objects by building larger perceptual units from local elements that are co-active together.

There is neurophysiological evidence consistent with these proposals. The Swiss researchers Von der Heydt, Peterhans and Baumgartner [11] used single cell electrophysiological recording and reported that cells in the primary visual cortex, area V1, responded to the presence of real contours but cells in the subsequent area V2 responded to an 'illusory contour' formed between two collinear, real contours (see Figure 4.7). That is, cells in area V2 seemed to respond on the basis of the relations between cells in V1 (e.g., firing when the V1 cells registered collinear edges – even if a real edge was not present and thus not detected in V1). Subsequently researchers have found responses to 'illusory' contours in V1 as well as V2 [12] and these results have also been confirmed when functional MRI has been used to measure brain activity [13]. Singer and Gray [14] have also noted that neurons responding to separate but collinear regions on a contour tend to fire together, which fits with the idea that co-activity in the neurons can be triggered when appropriate Gestalt properties are present in an image. More recent studies using fMRI in humans have chartered the process of learning to respond to Gestalt properties in stimuli, with a variety of different visual regions in

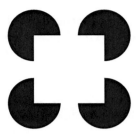

Figure 4.7 An example of an 'illusory contour'. When the pacmen are positioned to have collinear edges, then we can see an illusory contour joining the collinear edges to make a central square. Although there is no edge joining the pacmen, the brain responds as if an edge were present, presumably reflecting the fact that collinear edges tend to belong to a single contour in the real world. Von der Heydt and Peterhans proposed that this illusory contour was registered by neurons that pooled output from neurons responding to the collinear edges.

Source: Von der Heydt, R., Peterhans, E. and Baumgartner, G. (1984) Illusory contours and cortical neuron responses. *Science* 224: 1260–1262.

the brain responding more strongly to grouped elements as learning progresses [15]. This is consistent with the brain learning to put together local elements that co-occur with statistical regularity, to register the objects that determine these relations in the first place.

Are wholes more than the sum of their parts?

This parts-based approach can be contrasted with the view associated with another approach originating from Gestalt psychology and often associated with the phrase 'the whole is worth more than the sum of its parts' – a phrase suggesting that our perception of a whole stimulus is not simply based on summing together local, part elements. An example of where the whole seems to be more than the sum of the parts comes from experiments using stimuli such as those shown in Figure 4.8. In a now classic experiment, David Navon [16] presented observers with large letters (global shapes) made up of smaller letters (local shapes). The task was to respond to the identity of either the global shape (ignoring the local shapes) or the local shapes (ignoring the global shape) (e.g., is the local shape an S or an H?). Navon found that responses to the local shapes were affected by the identity of the global shapes – responses were fast if the global shape matched the local one and slow if the global shape called for the opposite response (H rather than S, as in Figure 4.8 left). This interference from the global shape should not arise if the global shape were coded by building it up from the local elements – we would identify the S before the H. Instead the results suggest that the global shape can be coded directly – without necessarily identifying the local elements first. One suggestion is that a global shape is coded directly at a relatively coarse level of resolution – this can be referred to as the low spatial frequency representation of the stimulus (Figure 4.8 right). For example, a low spatial frequency representation may be coded in parallel with any parts-based build-up of the global stimulus, and may even be coded more rapidly. The rapid coding of the low spatial frequency representation of a stimulus may result in the global stimulus taking precedence, influencing the identification response to a local element. The critical point here is that a low spatial frequency representation is not the sum of the parts, but a coarser representation that can be coded independently of parts-based processing.

Hierarchies, multi-modal processing, objects and scenes

Other important studies about how object processing, as opposed to feature processing, is achieved in the brain have been reported by Tanaka

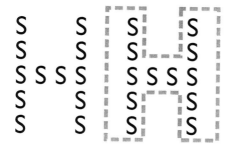

Figure 4.8 Left: a compound global letter made up of appropriately arranged local letters, as used originally by Navon. Right: interference from the global letter on the response to local letters suggests that a coarse representation of the global letter is coded directly by the brain. This is represented here by the grey dashed outline.

Source: Navon, D. (1977) Forest before trees: the precedence of global features in visual perception. *Cognitive Psychology* 9: 353–383.

et al. in Japan [17] and by Perrett and colleagues in Scotland [18]. Tanaka *et al.* [17] reported that, within the infero-temporal cortex of the monkey, cells respond to complex conjunctions (combinations) of features. Note that the infero-temporal cortex (area IT in Figure 4.2) is downstream from the early cortical regions studied by researchers such as Hubel and Wiesel. Cells in these downstream regions receive inputs from many cells in earlier cortical regions, and so are in a position to pool inputs from different kinds of features and from cells that respond to more local areas of a scene. This is consistent with the parts-based notion of a hierarchy of processes. The initial processes code individual features are in local regions and pass their activity onto cells at higher levels of the cortical visual stream, which respond to the conjunctive relations between features that define objects.

David Perrett followed up on an original finding by the American physiological psychologist Charlie Gross [19], who first documented the existence of cells in the superior part of the temporal lobe of the monkey that responded to faces more than other objects. This striking finding, of selective responding to particular classes of stimuli, suggests that the brain may have developed some degree of modularity – allocating neurons in some brain regions to particular classes of object, at least if those objects are very important to our survival (as can be argued for faces). We discuss the idea that there is a 'face processing module' in the brain later in this chapter and in more detail in Chapter 8 (What's in a face?). Perrett reported that there was a hierarchy of these face-coding cells. Neurons earlier in the pathway responded to a given face at a particular viewpoint, while cells further along the pathway showed a more invariant response across different facial viewpoints such as a face profile. Here it can be argued that the recognition of the same face across different views is achieved by pooling outputs from cells that initially respond to particular views. For example, a 'view invariant cell' may receive input from the different view-specific neurons for a given face, and so this cell is able to respond across different views (see Figure 4.9).

In studies of human vision there is also evidence for some populations of neurons responding in a view-specific manner while others respond in a view-invariant manner, firing to the same object irrespective of whether it appears in the same viewpoint. Vuilleumier and colleagues [20] used a technique known as fMRI adaptation to examine view-invariant responses in the ventral visual cortex. A very common property of neurons is that, having been initially activated by a stimulus, the same neuron will respond less strongly when the stimulus is repeatedly presented. This reduction in firing is known as adaptation and may reflect

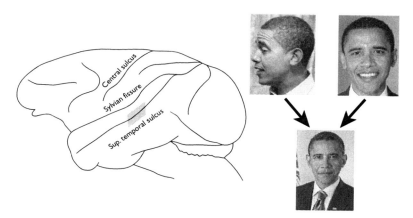

Figure 4.9 Left: the brain region where Perrett and colleagues recorded face-specific activity (in the superior temporal sulcus). Right: example of the proposed hierarchical activity in the superior temporal sulcus in which neurons responding to face seen from specific viewpoints feed through to 'canonical' neurons that respond irrespective of the specific viewpoint.

Source: Perrett, D. I., Hietanen, J. K., Oram, M. W. and Benson, P. J. (1992) Organization and functions of cells responsive to faces in the temporal cortex. *Philosophical Transactions of the Royal Society of London Series B – Biological Sciences* 335: 23–30.

the reduced novelty of repeated stimuli. Vuilleumier and colleagues found that cells in the ventral visual pathway in the left hemisphere showed reduced responses to the same stimulus irrespective of whether the stimulus appeared in the same or a different viewpoint. That is, cells in this part of the brain respond to a repeated object and not the viewpoint. In contrast, cells in the homologous region of the right hemisphere only showed adaptation when the viewpoint stayed the same. These authors conclude that different high-level ventral areas (e.g., in a structure called the fusiform gyrus which runs from the occipital to the temporal cortex) can show either view-specific or view-invariant responses, in the right and left hemispheres, Neurons in the right fusiform gyrus respond to specific views of objects while those in the left fusiform gyrus are less dependent on the specific view the object is seen from. This is not simply because the left hemisphere is important for language, with adaptation being shown because objects were assigned the same name. For example, the ventral visual areas showing adaptation to the same object did not show adaptation to different exemplars with the same name (e.g., to two different kinds of chair). Thus there appear to be visual 'recognition units' in the left hemisphere that respond across different views provided the same object is present. Whether the 'view-invariant' neurons in the left hemisphere receive input from the 'view-specific' neurons in the right hemisphere is not clear, though this would be the assumption of the hierarchical processing account.

Human object recognition not only shows invariance to changes in viewpoint but also to how the object is presented, for example, whether the object is shown as a photographic image or a line drawing, and whether (within limits!) some parts of the objects are obscured. While early visual regions (e.g., in area V1) can be differentially affected by whether a stimulus is presented as a photograph or line drawing, or whether it is occluded or not, an area in the occipital part of the ventral visual stream known as the 'Lateral Occipital Complex' (LOC) shows the same magnitude of response across the different ways that an object can be conveyed (e.g., whether as a photograph or a line drawing; whether partially covered or not), and neurons in this region demonstrate adaptation when the stimulus is initially shown in one manner even when subsequently presented in another (see Figure 4.10, Plate 4 in the plate section) [21]. These results fit the idea that the LOC performs a critical function in object recognition, enabling the same information to be registered no matter how the object is conveyed. Interestingly, there is also evidence [22] that the LOC not only responds to the *visual* appearance of objects but even to the same object presented in a different modality. For example, neurons in the LOC demonstrate adaptation from first feeling the shape of an object which affects the later response to the same object shown visually. Hence the LOC may be involved in responding to objects in a 'supra-modal manner', whether the objects are seen or felt.

If there is evidence for hierarchical processing of objects, from parts to wholes and from view-specific to view-invariant representations, then we can also ask whether our perception of a whole scene is built up in the same manner, for example, from coding the multiple objects that are present. Though there is evidence that fits with this general hierarchical account, other evidence suggests independent processing of scenes and objects – somewhat akin to the idea that global representations of objects can be coded independently of a parts-based process. Evidence consistent with scene recognition being built up from objects comes from studies with rudimentary visual scenes made up of pairs of objects. When these objects are positioned so that they appear to interact, then there is increased activation in the LOC and fusiform gyrus compared with when the objects do not appear to interact [23], suggesting that the neurons respond to the relationship formed between the objects and not just the individual objects. These data are consistent with a hierarchical coding account. On the other hand, other researchers [24] have reported that distinct neural regions are involved when objects and scenes are presented, with scenes recruiting cells in a medial region of the temporal cortex termed the parahippocampal cortex (while objects recruit cells in the LOC). For instance, while repeating the same objects in different background scenes leads to adaptation in occipital visual areas, repeating the background scenes but changing the objects produces adaptation in the parahippocampal region (see Figure 4.11, Plate 5 in the plate section). This engagement of different brain regions suggests that scenes are coded independently of the constituent objects and reflect instead, for instance, the presence of appropriate large-scale structural cues in the environment (e.g., the layout of critical landmarks). Scene recognition, like object recognition, may both be built up from constituent elements and coded from coarser representations of the whole stimulus (the object or the scene).

Interactions in object processing

Although we have stressed the role of hierarchical processing in visual object recognition, we should not think of the brain solely acting in a 'feed-forward' manner in which local parts are coded in greater wholes. There are at least as many feedback as feed-forward connections in the brain, and there is considerable evidence that feedback connections can modulate processing at earlier cortical levels. For example, Motter [25] studied a search task in which a monkey was cued to look for a target in a particular colour. It was found that activity in the colour area V4 was activated in a top-down manner by an expectation of the search target, biasing processing to favour the expected stimulus. In human vision, Schneider and Kastner [26], using fMRI, have shown that, when a target is expected, top-down projections not only lead to activity in the primarily visual area V1 in the cortex, but also to activity in sub-cortical structures such as the superior colliculus, which previously were assumed to operate purely in a stimulus-driven manner. Such top-down connections can enhance identification when objects are expected and may support the ability to image objects and to report their properties from memory. In cases such as John, the recognition of objects is typically facilitated if they are presented in a context and, as we shall review in Chapter 6, visual imagery for objects can even be preserved, despite the problem in stimulus-driven object recognition (e.g., when a stimulus is seen out of context). Such preserved abilities may depend on top-down projections being initially present.

From what to where to action!

So far we have stressed the processes that support the process of object recognition – that tell us what an object is. However, this covers only one (albeit important) aspect of what vision does. There is also a large amount of research indicating that, outside of the ventral pathway, visually-responsive neurons perform other jobs. In particular, neurons in the dorsal (occipital-parietal) pathway respond to properties that determine how we directly interact with the world – such as when we reach and grasp objects. We have already noted the distinction between 'ventral' and 'dorsal' visual processing made by Ungerleider and Mishkin [6], who argued that the ventral visual pathway computes 'what' a stimulus is while the dorsal visual pathway codes 'where' stimuli are in the world. The distinction made by Ungerleider and Mishkin from animal studies has been supported by brain imaging work with humans. For example, Courtney and colleagues [27] had people remember either individual faces or the locations on a screen where the faces fell, and measured brain activity using PET. They found that memory for faces was associated with activation of ventral regions in the occipital and temporal cortices, as well as regions in the right frontal cortex (right Figure 4.12) likely involved in memorising rather than visually processing the faces. In contrast, memory for location was linked to activity in the posterior parietal cortex, consistent with the Ungerleider and Mishkin account [6].

There is evidence too for the involvement of the dorsal visual stream in coding where objects are in depth as well as in 2D space. An example comes from a study by Berryhill and Olson [28]. These authors presented participants with images of objects seen from different depths and the task was to determine whether each object belonged in the kitchen. Although it was not relevant to the main task, consecutive objects could fall at the same or at different depths, and 'adaptation' could be measured when the objects stayed at the same depth compared with when they varied in depth. Depth adaptation was shown in area V3/V3A, in the posterior part of the dorsal visual stream. Interestingly, Berryhill and Olson also reported a patient (patient 'EE 555') whose lesion overlapped with the brain area which adapted to depth in normal observers (see Figure 4.13, Plate 6 in the plate section). This patient was able to judge whether objects belonged in the kitchen but was impaired at judging the

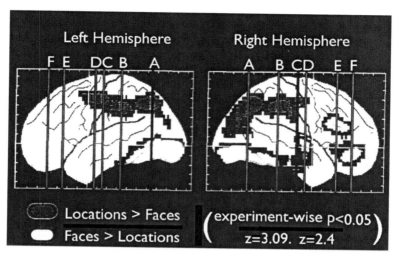

Figure 4.12 See p. 36. Areas marked in black on the outline brains represent regions where there was increased activation when memory was for location rather than for individual faces, while areas circled in white represent areas more active for face memory than for memory for locations. Area A is towards the back of the brain and area F towards the front.

Source: From Courtney, S. M., Ungeleider, L. G., Keil, K. and Haxby, J. V. (1996) Object and spatial visual working memory activate separate neural systems in human cortex. *Cerebral Cortex* 6: 39–49, by permission of Oxford University Press.

relative depths of objects (Figure 4.13 bottom). The results from normal observers and from the patient are complementary. It appears that the posterior part of the dorsal visual stream codes depth, so that depth perception is impaired when the brain region is damaged.

The location and depth information coded within the dorsal stream not only enables us to know where objects are but it also enables us to act upon them, since any action we make to an object is contingent on our computing where the object is (in depth as well as lateral distance). Again we can call upon evidence from brain imaging to illustrate this. Culham and colleagues measured brain activity using fMRI when participants either grasped or pointed to an object placed in front of them [29]. They also measured brain activity to intact and scrambled pictures of objects. The contrast between intact and scrambled images of objects activated area LOC in the ventral visual stream, which we have already noted responds to integrated parts of objects (e.g., even when some parts are occluded). In contrast, the comparison between grasping and reaching led to increased activity in parts of the posterior parietal cortex. The different brain regions activated by grasping as opposed to reaching, and by the presence of intact as opposed to scrambled parts of objects, are shown in Figure 4.14 (Plate 7 in the plate section). The critical role of the posterior parietal cortex in grasping objects has been one of the pieces of evidence leading researchers to argue that the dorsal stream not only codes object locations but also is critical for using visual information to direct action to objects. We consider this argument in more detail in Chapter 9.

Modularity in vision: processing faces

It can be argued that, of all the visual objects that we are able to recognise, faces are perhaps the most visually complex and most similar to other members of the same categories. Faces – perhaps more than other stimuli – are also socially important, enabling us to recognise friends and family. Due to the high visual demands of face processing, and the social imperative to use faces to individuate people, the brain may have developed special-purpose processes to serve face recognition, which may not be demanded when other objects are recognised. This is a controversial proposal that has its support in evidence showing that face recognition is disproportionately affected by certain visual manipulations. For example, individuals are very difficult to recognise when seen from upside down (when their faces are inverted), whereas inversion tends not to have such a drastic effect on other objects. Consider Figure 4.15 [30]. If you look at the top two images of inverted faces you can notice that they differ to some degree, but the differences are only apparent if you scrutinise the images. Now look at the bottom two images of upright faces. Suddenly the differences between the images are striking – yet these are the same images as the top ones, but rotated into their normal upright orientation! The striking contrast between the saliency of the feature changes in upright and inverted faces indicates that face recognition is, to some degree, tuned to seeing faces that are in their standard, upright orientation. Also, when faces are seen in an upright orientation we seem much more sensitive to the spatial relations between their features (e.g., the positions of the eyes relative to the eyebrows) than when faces are inverted. This marked sensitivity is consistent with face processing being highly dependent on coding the spatial relations between facial features. This is often referred to as 'configural coding' – where recognition

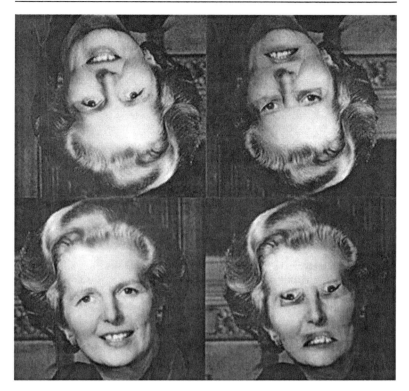

Figure 4.15 The different effects of scrambling the positions and orientations of facial features (the eyes, eyebrows and mouth) when faces are inverted (top) and when upright (bottom). The manipulation of the features is much more salient when faces are upright relative to when they are inverted. This particular manipulation, of inverting local facial features in inverted vs. upright faces is known as 'Thatcherisation', since the original study demonstrated the effect using images of Margaret Thatcher.

Source: From Thompson, P. (1980) Margaret Thatcher: a new illusion. *Perception* 9: 483–484. Courtesy of Pion Ltd, London, www.envplan.com.

depends not just on the presence of particular features but also on how the features are spatially positioned in relation to one another.

One example of configural coding was presented by Takane and Sergent [31], using stimuli we later borrowed for experiments of face processing on John (see Chapter 8). Takane and Sergent had people judge whether two faces were identical or differed. When the faces differed,

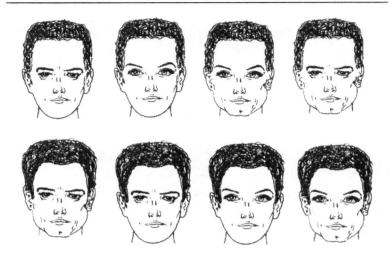

Figure 4.16 Stimuli used by Takane and Sergent (1983). The faces each have one of two hairstyles, noses and chins. A pair of faces was presented and observers had to decide if the faces were identical or differed. Performance was much more efficient if all three features differed relative to if just one or two differed.

Source: Takane, Y. and Sergent, J. (1983) Multidimensional scaling models for reaction times and same-different judgements. *Psychometrika* 48: 393–423.

they could have an alternative hairstyle, a different nose or a different mouth – or any combination of these differences (see Figure 4.16). Tanake and Sergent tested whether the data could be explained by assuming there was independent processing of each of the features and concluded that it could not. For example, responses when the faces differed in three features could not be explained in terms of the speed to respond to differences in single or pairs of features – faces differing in three features could be discriminated much more easily than when fewer differences were present. The results were taken to suggest that we respond to more than the presence of facial features and we are sensitive to the spatial relations between the features – what we will refer to as the facial configuration. The configural relations between the features change as more features differ, making it easier to perceive differences between the faces.

There is considerable evidence too for face processing being relatively specialised in the human brain. For example, studies of brain imaging have consistently shown that, when we view faces compared with other objects, there is increased activation in a cluster of regions which may perform different functions when faces are processed (e.g., the so-called occipital and fusiform face areas, along with the superior temporal sulcus) (see Figure 4.17 in the plate section). For example, Liu and colleagues carried out two manipulations [32]. They varied whether faces did or did not have their normal internal parts (eyes, nose and mouth), and they varied whether or not the internal elements occupied standard spatial positions for a face (see Figure 4.18). They measured brain activity using

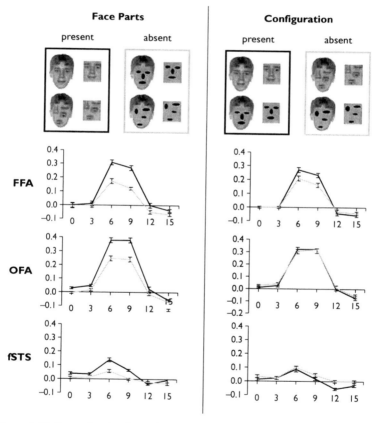

Figure 4.18 Example stimuli used by Lui and colleagues (2010). The face parts (eyes, nose and mouth) were present or absent (left), and the spatial configuration of the features was either present or absent (right).

Source: From Liu, J., Harris, A. and Kanwisher, N. (2010) Perception of face parts and face configurations: an fMRI study. *Journal of Cognitive Neuroscience* 22: 203–211. Reprinted by permission of MIT Press Journals.

fMRI and noted differences between the occipital (OFA) and superior temporal (fSTS) areas, on the one hand, and the fusiform face area (FFA), on the other. All three areas showed a greater response when the face parts were present than when they were obscured, indicating sensitivity to the individual features of faces. However, the OFA and fSTS did not differentiate between face elements in normal and in scrambled spatial locations, while the FFA did. This is consistent with the FFA in particular responding to the spatial relations between the features (i.e., to a configural property of faces), over and above responses to the features.

Pitcher and colleagues [33] extended this further by measuring brain activity to static and moving faces. While the OFA and FFA regions did not respond differentially to static and moving faces, fSTS did – showing an enhanced response when faces moved. They linked this result to the role of the fSTS in processing 'biological motion' – that is, patterns of

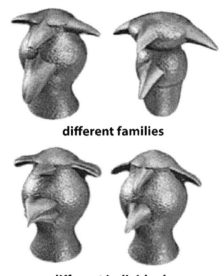

different families

different individuals

Figure 4.19   Examples of stimuli known as 'Greebles'. Essentially these are items constructed using similar parts but re-arranged to create items which can vary as individuals around a general 'family' of Greebles, which have common features.

Source: Gauthier, I. *et al.* (1999) Activation in the middle fusiform 'face area' increases with expertise in recognising novel objects. *Nature Neuroscience* 2: 568–573. Reprinted by permission from Macmillan Publishers Ltd.

movement as conveyed by moving organisms. The findings suggest that not only are there several brain areas that are selectively activated by faces, but these regions may also carry out different tasks – with some (e.g., the fSTS) especially responsive to dynamic changes in faces, as may occur when we encounter people in social contexts.

A controversial point is whether these brain regions activated by faces respond in a highly selective way – just to faces – or not. For example Gauthier, Tarr and colleagues have reported that when people learn to discriminate non-face stimuli that come from visually homogeneous sets of items ('Greebles'; see Figure 4.19), then there is activation of similar brain regions to those activated by faces [34]. But does this mean that faces are not special, or does it mean that Greebles are processed like faces? One way to test the specificity of the brain's response to faces is to assess if there can be very selective losses of face processing after brain damage. We return to this point in Chapter 8.

Visual words

In addition to showing a relatively selective response to faces, the brain also shows selectivity in responding to visually presented words. Figure 4.20, (see plate section) illustrates activity recorded using fMRI when observers saw different symbols – familiar words, letter strings with frequently co-occurring groups of letters (quadrigrams and bigrams – so called because they had sets of either four or two consecutive letters which occur frequently together), frequent letters, infrequent letters (e.g., JZWY) and 'false font items' (letter-like symbols) [35]. The upper brains in Figure 4.20 are seen from below, in the bottom right section there is a side view of the left hemisphere (the occipital lobe, containing visually-responsive neurons, shown to the right). The top right brain indicates activity to words (in red), relative to when there was a blank screen. In the following brains in the same row, the response to the other symbols (relative to the blank screen) is plotted, with new colours added (from yellow down to purple) according to the reduced level of activity for those stimuli relative to words. Note that, in the left hemisphere, there is considerable differentiation between the conditions, starting from the most anterior regions which are selectively activated by words to the more posterior regions which respond to several classes of stimuli. For example, false fonts and unrelated letters create minimal activity in the most anterior regions (shown in purple), while bigrams reduce activity in these anterior areas (depicted in yellow and green). The side view of the left hemisphere indicates the different effects of letters and letter-like stimuli, as activity is traced from posterior to more anterior regions of the ventral visual areas.

The differential response to words is particularly evident in the fusiform gyrus in the left hemisphere, and it has been proposed that this brain region acts as a 'visual word form system', supporting the visual recognition of words [36]. The system shows a graded response according to the visual similarity of the stimulus to known words with more activity for the more word-like stimuli. Interestingly, this same region of ventral cortex increases in its activity as individuals learn to read [37] suggesting that its relatively modular response to words is subject to learning.

Conclusion

The work we have reviewed here illustrates something of the complexity of visual processing in the brain. The brain decomposes images into local elements and reconstructs representations of more global objects using laws based on the statistical regularities of our environment. There can also be direct coding of global forms and scenes. There is some specialisation not only for coding basic features such as colour, motion and depth, but also for coding more complex stimuli, such as scenes, faces and words. Given that these processes are also localised in different brain areas, it is not surprising that individuals can suffer selective losses of particular visual processes if there is selective damage to one of these areas. In John's case, the damage affected several regions in the ventral visual stream, on both sides of his brain. The effects of these lesions on particular aspects of visual processing provide important insights into how those processes operate in the brain.

Chapter 5

A short history of visual agnosia

A dog and a cow appeared alike, but on seeing a cow he would know it could not be a dog, because a dog could not be that size.

[38]

Armed with information about how visual processing operates in the brain, we can now consider how investigators have thought about visual agnosia – the loss of visual recognition after brain damage. The study of visual recognition disorders has a long history. Some of the first reports came from experiments where animals had visual regions of the brain lesioned to assess if these central changes would induce cortical blindness. One striking observation was made by Munk in 1881 [39]. Munk noticed that partial ablation of visual cortex in a dog produced a marked drop in the animal's responsiveness to familiar objects but the dog was not blind – it was able to negotiate its environment without bumping into obstacles. Munk suggested that the dog could 'see' the objects but not 'recognise' them. He argued that the brain lesion disrupted 'memory images' acquired by previous experience, so that, as a consequence, the animal perceived stimuli that were stripped of their meaning, so to speak. However, given that the animal remained able to walk around objects, the loss of recognition for 'what' the object was did not lead to poor coding of 'where' the object was.

Lissauer's framework

The proposal put forward by Munk pre-dated some similar ideas promoted by the German neurologist Lissauer [40]. Lissauer is often credited with putting forward the first theoretical account of visual agnosia. He described the case of an 80-year-old salesman who had experienced a blow to his head subsequent to which his visual recognition abilities were severely impaired while his ability to 'see' apparently remained unaffected. Lissauer diagnosed the condition as 'Seelenblindheit', or mind blindness. There had been earlier descriptions of similar cases. Wilbrand [41] applied the term 'psychic blindness' to a patient with a similar impairment and (interestingly) Freund [42] coined the term agnosia to describe a disorder of visual recognition which could not be accounted for by impairments in basic sensory processes (e.g., deficits in visual acuity), or to intellectual deterioration. Lissauer suggested that visual recognition required two distinct processing stages: the first (*apperception*) was described as 'the stage of conscious awareness of a sensory impression'. The second, *associative* stage demanded access to concepts related to the object – that is, to stored memories. Taking as an example a violin, Lissauer stressed the wealth of different sensory associations that can be built into our memories – the image of the object, its sound, its name, our tactile experience of handling it, the context in which it might typically visually appear. The specific nature of memories and associations for any object will of course vary between individuals but nonetheless most people will have a rich concept for each object they know, based on this distribution of associations. Using his two-stage framework, Lissauer suggested that two different forms of agnosia could be distinguished: an *apperceptive agnosia*, where there is poor assimilation of the perceptual features of objects; and an *associative agnosia*, where the apperceptive stage is preserved but associative knowledge fails to be activated normally. This associative problem could come about either because there is a disconnection of associative knowledge from the features coded at the apperceptive stage, or because associative knowledge itself is damaged. This last idea is strikingly close to Munk's [39] interpretation of the behaviour of his agnosic dog.

Lissauer not only provided a conceptual framework for understanding visual recognition disorders, he also proposed methods for distinguishing the putative deficits, by testing: (1) shape discrimination; and (2) shape copying in patients. He reported the results of both tests with his patient GL. For shape discrimination, GL was initially asked to detect obvious differences between simple shapes, followed by minimal differences between more complex shapes. GL performed well with the simple tests but not with the more complex stimuli. From these observations Lissauer argued that perceptual abilities may lie on a continuum, from the computation of simple shape features through to the coding of more complex representations. Given his problem with the more complex shapes, we might speculate that GL's problem was at this intermediate process of coding complex shapes, but not in computing simple features. Although GL struggled with complex shape discriminations, he was able to copy objects. From this last result Lissauer suggested that GL was a case of associative agnosia, but, given the problem that GL had with complex shapes, Lissauer was also sceptical that 'pure' associative agnosia could exist, without the patient having some form of contributing perceptual problem.

Does associative agnosia exist?

Visual agnosia is an extremely uncommon disorder and led a number of eminent scientists to doubt its existence in quite a forcible way! For instance, in a paper published in the journal *Brain* in 1972, Bender and Feldman [43] stated:

> A review of our case records in the Department of Neurology at the Mount Sinai Hospital for the past twenty years failed to disclose a single case of so-called visual agnosia without concomitant defects in the fields of vision or perception, mental dysfunction, or dysphasia. In every patient who showed inability to recognize a common object visually, though able to do so by touch or by sound, there were also alterations in vision, and often in other sensory functions and in mentation.

After grouping all their cases, they report a spectrum had emerged with patients having severe mental and mild visual defects at one end and mild mental and severe visual defects at the other: there were a variety of combinations of the visual disorders in the middle. An influential British neurologist, Critchley, further stated that 'Cases of visual agnosia, though a commonplace in medical text-books, represent – let us admit – an extreme rarity in clinical practice. The validity of most of the handful of recorded cases is indeed open to serious criticism. [44]. Critchley went so far as to state: 'Unless one holds mental reservation about "agnosia", neurology would be better off without that particular term.'

While some doubted whether the disorder actually existed, others tried to provide an explanation for the patterns of performance observed in the patients; for instance, Bay [45] suggested that standard clinical tests of visual function were insufficiently sensitive to detect deficits that may play a significant role in recognition impairments. In particular, he argued that while standard measures of visual detection can chart whether there is central or peripheral loss of visual field, they do not assess the differential sensitivity/functions of the different areas of the field. Furthermore, standard assessments do not include measurement of visual thresholds, or the effects of prolonged stimulation. Bay applied a range of visual sensory assessments to a number of patients including one patient with a frank recognition disturbance (Case 8). The patient, a 60-year-old man with congenital amblyopia of the right eye, suddenly developed a failure in the ability to visually recognise objects. He awoke from an afternoon nap to find that he could not identify the clothes on the table in front of him, nor his neighbours in the street (including his daughter) when he went out for a walk. On assessment (of the left eye) the following day, eye movements, acuity and visual field were all within normal limits; however, he showed a marked impairment in the recognition of visual objects and pictures. Bay stated: 'As far as I know of the literature, he is the only case of object agnosia with normal visual acuity and fields and with no mental deterioration.' Measures of the patient's visual fields were initially conducted in full daylight; however, if the lighting was reduced, the patient's visual field contracted while that of a normal control remained constant. Bay used this result to account for the patient's recognition deficit. He stated: 'We find a heavy impairment of the sensory activity which fully explains the gnostic (recognition) disturbances. That means that there is no need for any specific disorders of gnosis on the psychological level in the classical sense of agnosia.' That is, the argument was that a sensory loss could account for the recognition disorder without falling back on the idea of a higher-order problem in accessing stored object knowledge. A contemporary of Bay, George Ettlinger [46] set out to test Bay's hypothesis. He carried out a careful assessment of the sensory status in small groups of patients without either field losses or perceptual defects, with field losses but without perceptual defects or with both field and perceptual deficits. He tested several aspects of perception: acuity when stimuli were briefly presented; the rate at which flickering lights fuse into a stable, non-flickering stimulus; brightness discrimination; acuity for small objects; movement perception, and whether there was abnormal adaptation/fading after prolonged stimulus exposure. Sensory deficits were demonstrated in patients both with and without visual field loss but, critically, sensory deficits were not greater in those with visual field loss. Ettlinger argued that sensory status alone could not explain the presence or absence of a recognition disorder. A point raised by Ettlinger himself, however, was that he had not included anyone with frank visual agnosia. At a later date, though, Ettlinger and Wyke did assess a patient with a pure visual agnosia and, again, while there was evidence of sensory loss (e.g., reduced brightness discrimination), the problems were no worse than those found in non-agnosic individuals [47]. However, this patient did show some confusion about where they were, and when the actual testing took place. Ettlinger and Wyke 'concluded that confusion, together with a visual defect, caused a deficit resembling visual agnosia'.

In contrast to these arguments within human neuropsychology, studies in the monkey conducted in the 1960s showed that lesions of the cortical regions receiving direct input from vision produce abnormal sensory performance (e.g., in the time taken for flickering visual stimuli to fuse into a single event) but little impairment in visual form discrimination [48]. On the other hand, animals with lesions further along the visual pathway in the brain (in inferotemporal regions, see Figure 4.2) can have impaired form discrimination without associated problems in sensory discrimination [49].

Additional emerging data from human cases highlight that not all agnosias are caused by perceptual impairment and also that access to different types of stored knowledge can be distinguished. At the same time that we began testing John, we also worked with another patient, JB, who had impaired object recognition after sustaining a head injury [50]. We tested object recognition by giving JB sets of three objects, two of which would be used together with the third being from the same general category but not used directly with the others, e.g., a knife, a fork and a whisk. JB was poor at picking out the two he would use together (scoring about 55 per cent correct). However, the task presented no problem when he was given the names of the objects (scoring 100 per cent correct). This poor visual recognition of which objects should be used together contrasted with JB's performance on other tasks where access to different types of stored knowledge was tested. An example comes from a study of 'object decision' where JB was required to discriminate drawings of real objects from those of 'nonobjects'. The difficulty of the object decision varies with how similar the nonobjects are to real objects; the more similar the nonobject, the more the task demands access to precise visual knowledge about objects.

For the test with JB we created nonobjects by putting together the parts of two objects that came from the same category, and that made a shape similar to other members of that category (see Figure 5.1). The task was sufficiently taxing that even control participants made some errors. Despite this, JB performed as well as controls – he accepted the real objects and rejected even plausible nonobjects as incorrect. As he carried out the task he remarked that some of the stimuli looked very familiar to him (the real objects) and others did not (the nonobjects). The results suggest that JB was able to perform the task based on access to stored knowledge which told him how visually familiar the stimuli were, even though he was then impaired at accessing full 'conceptual' knowledge about which objects can be used together – indicated by his poor performance at judging which objects go with one another. This pattern of performance, in which patients succeed at object decision but remain impaired at accessing conceptual knowledge about objects, has subsequently been reported in a number of patients [e.g., 51]. The dissociation between accessing perceptual and conceptual knowledge suggests that we need to distinguish between different types of stored knowledge involved in object recognition – perceptual knowledge about the shape and perhaps other visual features of an object being distinct from conceptual knowledge about how objects function, where they are found, and so forth (see Figure 5.2). It is certainly difficult to argue that such patients have a fundamental problem in processing the perceptual properties of objects, given that they 'pass' the difficult object decision test (where control participants too can make errors) but 'fail' an associative matching task from vision which can be accomplished easily when stimuli are presented in another modality. To our mind, such cases present perhaps the clearest evidence that associative agnosia can exist.

Other evidence for agnosia occurring sometimes after normal perceptual processing brings us back to Elizabeth Warrington's work on

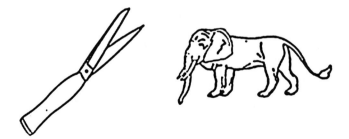

Figure 5.1 Example nonobjects for an object decision test. The task requirement is to decide whether each stimulus is a real object or a nonobject. With nonobjects created to have plausible properties of objects, the task requires access to stored knowledge of the object's structure but not necessarily to stored information about the semantic or associative properties of objects, nor to its name.

Source: From Riddoch, M. J. and Humphreys, G. W. (1993) *BORB: Birmingham Object Recognition Battery*. Hove: Psychology Press, reprinted by permission of the publisher (Taylor & Francis Group, http://www.informaworld.com).

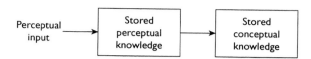

Figure 5.2 A simple theoretical framework distinguishing between different forms of stored knowledge that needs to be accessed to achieve object recognition

'unusual views'. In Chapter 1 we mentioned that we started out by examining the work of Elizabeth Warrington on the recognition of objects in 'unusual views'. Warrington had shown that patients with damage to posterior parietal cortex had problems in recognising stimuli appearing in unusual views [1]. An example of an 'unusual views' matching task is presented in Figure 5.3. These problems with unusual views were noted particularly in patients who had sustained right hemisphere brain damage. Patients with left parietal damage passed on tasks of unusual view matching but then had difficulty at matching objects that were used to achieve

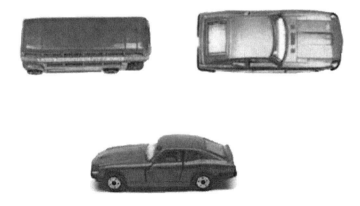

Figure 5.3 Example stimuli from an unusual-view matching test. The task is to decide which of the two top pictures is the same as the object depicted in the bottom picture. In the top image, the target (the car) is rotated to appear in an unusual view (seen from the top). Patients with right parietal damage can be impaired at this matching task.

Source: From Humphreys, G. W. and Riddoch, M. J. (2006) Features, objects, actions: the cognitive neuropsychology of visual object processing. *Cognitive Neuropsychology* 23: 156–183, reprinted by permission of the publisher (Taylor & Francis Group, http://www.informaworld.com).

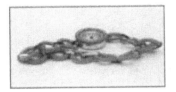
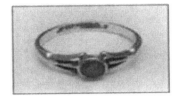
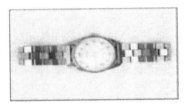

Figure 5.4 Example 'function match' stimuli. Patients are required to judge which of the top two items is the same kind of object as the bottom stimulus. Patients with impaired object recognition can fail on this task despite succeeding at difficult unusual view matches (Figure 5.3), suggesting that the task requires access to forms of conceptual knowledge beyond perceptual coding of the stimuli.

Source: From Humphreys, G. W. and Riddoch, M. J. (2006) Features, objects, actions: the cognitive neuropsychology of visual object processing. *Cognitive Neuropsychology* 23: 156–183, reprinted by permission of the publisher (Taylor & Francis Group, http://www.informaworld.com).

the same function – even when these objects were shown in standard views (see Figure 5.4). Warrington suggested that the patients with left hemisphere damage had spared perceptual processing but poor access to conceptual information about what objects are used for. Other studies have also gone on to present data from patients who could perform unusual view matching while having impaired access to stored information about object, including failing on difficult object decision tasks (our index of access to stored perceptual knowledge; Figure 5.2) [52]. Again this is a pattern consistent with Lissauer's definition of associative agnosia in which there is poor access to object meaning but intact perception. In the latter case, perceptual processing is sufficient to sustain matching across unusual views but there is subsequently impaired access to stored perceptual knowledge about objects.

Views of apperceptive agnosia

Unlike the arguments about associative agnosia, there have been fewer doubts that apperceptive agnosia exists, where patients have poor object recognition due to impaired perceptual processes. Nevertheless, there have been different views about the nature of the perceptual impairments. One of the historical limitations with the field was that many of the initial cases were described anecdotally, and there was a lack of theoretically-motivated testing of the different processes that make up visual perception. A good example is a case study reported by Macrae and Trolle [38] whose patient presented with very similar symptoms to John. For example, the quote with which we started the chapter could almost have come from John, as the patient used logical deduction to work out what an object was – eliminating alternative possibilities rather than apprehending the object's identity at a glance. When asked to describe how he saw faces, Macrae and Trolle's patient stated:

> I see the whole face—the bit I am looking at (pointing with his fore-finger to a spot on the questioner's chin) is quite clear—I see every single hair quite clearly—but everything else is different, as though there was a thin layer over it all, or as though it were out of focus.

From these answers Macrae and Trolle concluded that the patient only saw detail in a very small area of central vision, and had low resolution processing elsewhere. The small area of high detailed processing was proposed to cause the apperceptive agnosia.

Subsequent to Macrae and Trolle's work, investigators began to develop more systematic analyses. Efron developed a very simple test in which the patient is presented with squares and rectangles which are matched in brightness but differ in shape [53]. The task requires the patient to discriminate the squares from the rectangles (Figure 5.5). The first application of this test to an agnostic patient was carried out by Benson and Greenberg in 1969 [54]. They found that the patient per-formed poorly on the task and argued that there was a basic problem in assimilating the two dimensions that make up shapes. They proposed

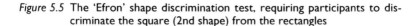

Figure 5.5 The 'Efron' shape discrimination test, requiring participants to dis-criminate the square (2nd shape) from the rectangles

that this problem in computing form was key to the apperceptive deficit. Deficits in the 'Efron discrimination task' have subsequently been reported in other apperceptive agnostics, and have become a defining symptom of what has been termed 'form agnosia' [55].

Benson and Greenberg's agnostic patient suffered carbon monoxide poisoning which can lead to small disseminated brain lesions, often not confined to a single brain region. Campion and Latto [56] seized on this point and put forward an alternative view of why such patients fail on the 'Efron task'. These investigators argued that small disseminated lesions in the visual cortex of carbon monoxide patients could introduce small blind spots through the visual field, which would in turn disrupt the ability to assimilate shape information. According to Campion and Latto, the visual field loss in these patients was the prime cause of their problems in object recognition, not the process of computing shape itself.

In contrast to these views of apperceptive agnosia as either a problem in resolution across a small spatial area (the idea of Macrae) or a problem in basic shape perception (as argued by Benson and Greenburg and also Campion and Latto, though for different reasons), Elizabeth Warrington proposed that apperceptive agnosia was in fact the problem in unusual view recognition that she had documented in patients with damage to the right parietal cortex [1, 57]. This argument was put forward because such patients do not suffer a basic sensory deficit but still have problems at an intermediate stage of visual processing, prior to access to stored knowledge taking place. Patients with poor recognition of objects in unusual views show poor invariance in visual processing, meaning that their recognition is not invariant to the changes in viewpoint that we can normally cope with. If the problems in invariance extended beyond the case of viewpoint change to include poor recognition when there are changes in lighting, stimulus size and depth – the conditions that we might well encounter in the real world – then a problem in computing invariant information could contribute to poor recognition even for objects in standard views (especially with non-standard lighting, changed size, and so forth). In contrast, for patients with problems in shape perception on the Efron test, the contribution of a sensory impairment cannot be excluded.

Of course, this argument raises questions about what other processes may take place between sensory coding and the basic assimilation of simple two-dimensional shape, and, on the other hand, the perceptual encoding of more complex objects (e.g., where multiple parts need to be integrated and segmented from parts belonging to other complex stimuli in scenes). Our review in Chapter 4 indicated that the brain must carry out multiple processes between sensory coding and object recognition in order for us to perceive and recognise objects. John suffered brain damage to just these processes, and, as we now go on to describe, his case helps us understand how the processes take place.

Conclusion

The history of studies of agnosia is mixed, and, perhaps due to the rarity of the disorder, clinicians have been sceptical about whether a 'pure' problem in recognition can occur without the patient having some form of lower-level perceptual or sensory loss. Clearly it is important to try and establish whether sensory loss is a contributory factor in a patient. The work also demonstrates that there can be dissociations between various stages of recognition – the basic coding of shape, the ability to compute object representations that are invariant to viewpoint, the ability to access different forms of stored information (about learned perceptual and conceptual knowledge). These dissociations provide a skeleton framework to guide our analysis of John's perceptual abilities.

Chapter 6

Integrative agnosia

I can see the details but I don't get an impression of how they relate.

(John)

The background to our starting out to test John was confused. Did visual agnosia exist outside of any basic perceptual or sensory impairment? If there was a perceptual impairment, what was the critical factor (poor discrimination outside the area of central vision, poor shape discrimination, a lack of invariance in processing)? A starting place was to assess basic aspects of his perception using some the standard 'markers' of performance – the Efron shape test, copying objects, matching objects across unusual views, performing object decisions, and so forth.

An initial diagnosis using standard tests

As indicated in Chapter 3, John was very accurate at copying, as illustrated by his reproduction of the etching of St Paul's cathedral (Figure 3.2) [58]. He was also good at the Efron shape-matching task (Figure 5.5). Given a simple, regular two-dimensional shape, he could discriminate at a normal level whether it was a square or a rectangle [59]. He was also well able to perform particular 'unusual views' tasks – notably if some of the features present in one image of an object could be matched to the same features in the other image (an example might be the marks on the bonnet of the car, in Figure 5.3) [60]. Given the history of studies of agnosia, good performance on the Efron shape-matching task, accurate copying and the ability to carry out unusual view matching could be taken to indicate that visual perception is operating normally. Most impressively, John could also perform other demanding perceptual tasks extremely well. Figure 6.1 shows two sets of patches composed of

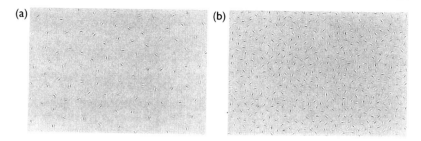

Figure 6.1 A test of sensitivity to grouping between the aligned (collinear) 'Gabor' elements, John was able to detect the circular pattern in both the left ((a), easy) and right ((b), hard) displays. John performed at the top end of a group of age-matched control participants.

Source: From Giersch, A., Humphreys, G. W., Boucart, M. and Koviáks, I. (2000) The computation of occluded contours in visual agnosia: evidence of early computation prior to shape binding and figure-ground coding. *Cognitive Neuropsychology* 17: 731–759, reprinted by permission of the publisher (Taylor & Francis Group, http://www.informaworld.com).

oriented line elements at particular spatial frequencies (widths of pattern). Within each array one set of patches is aligned to create a circle shape. To see this shape your visual system needs to group the local patches to form the closed shape. The task can be made arbitrarily difficult by introducing more and more patches at random orientations so that it becomes impossible for anyone to systematically detect the pattern target. We examined where this threshold fell for John compared with control participants similar in age. The left side display (a) contains a pattern in its bottom left corner which is relatively easy to detect. The right side display (b) contains a pattern in its lower right corner but this is much more difficult to detect due to the increased number of distractors present. The pattern on the right represents John's detection threshold – the maximum level of distraction where he could still detect the grouped shape. This level was, if anything, rather better than the level achieved by the control participants [61]!

Alongside his good performance on some of these tests of 'low-level' visual perception, John was also able look at a display of visual elements and code the 'average' information present. We presented him with displays of oriented elements and he had to detect whether the majority of items were oriented to the left or right of the vertical. This task is easy when all the elements have the same orientation but it becomes increasingly difficult as the items themselves vary in orientation (see Figure 6.2). By varying the orientations of the items, you can measure the threshold

Figure 6.2 In (a), all of the elements have the same orientation, to the left of vertical. In (b), the orientations of the individual elements vary, making it much more difficult to decide whether the average orientation falls to the left or right of vertical.

Source: Reprinted from Allen, H. A., Humphreys, G. W. and Bridge, H. (2007) Ventral extra-striate cortical areas are required for optimal orientation averaging. *Vision Research* 47: 766–775, with permission from Elsevier.

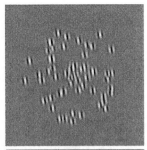

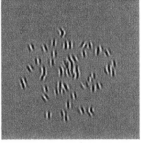

when performance breaks down – when the average orientation can no longer be computed. John's threshold for judging the average orientation of the elements did not differ from that of controls [62].

In contrast to his good performance on these tasks requiring perceptual judgements, John was consistently impaired in his ability to access stored information about objects. He was impaired at naming objects from vision – despite being perfectly able to generate the correct name when given a verbal definition rather than the picture of an object, and despite being good at naming objects from touch. Note here that naming to a verbal definition and naming from touch can be the more difficult tasks for normal participants. John was also poor at carrying out object decision tasks, where the requirement is only to judge whether an object is more familiar than a non-object. Some agnosics are able to perform object decision tasks even though they have poor access to conceptual knowledge about objects (e.g., patient JB described in Chapter 5). These results indicate that John had a visual *recognition* impairment, so that he was poor at accessing stored perceptual as well as conceptual knowledge about objects [58].

At first glance then it is tempting to conclude that John's recognition problem did not reflect a perceptual deficit. He seemed able to assimilate the basic shape of objects; he could group elements based on their local aligned edges (Figure 6.1) and he could compute the average of a set of orientations (Figure 6.2). We have also noted that John showed good long-term memory for the properties of objects he was unable to identify. He could draw objects from memory (Figure 3.3) and he could give accurate descriptions of the visual properties of objects. Stored memory of objects appeared intact. It follows that John's impairment is caused by the normally processed perceptual information failing to match his intact stored object knowledge. In Lissauer's terminology, John can be labelled an associative agnosic.

This argument can be called a 'disconnection account' of agnosia. The argument is that there is not a problem with either forming perceptual representations or accessing conceptual representations of objects, but rather the two forms of representation have been disconnected through a brain lesion [63]. Disconnection accounts of agnosia have been made before – mostly based on the argument that the anatomical connections between brain areas have been damaged, so that one region cannot communicate with another [61]. This can be illustrated by considering the case of patient JB, whom we discussed in Chapter 5. JB was impaired at both naming and making 'conceptual' judgements to objects based upon the objects being used together [50]. In contrast to this poor 'recognition' performance, JB carried out difficult object decision tasks at a normal level, discriminating between drawings of real objects and images of plausible non-objects (Figure 5.1). He also had good knowledge of the conceptual relations between objects when given their names To account for the results, we proposed a form of disconnection account whereby JB had spared access to stored perceptual knowledge from vision, and access to conceptual knowledge from object names, but there was a disconnection between these two forms of stored representation (see Figure 6.3). John's case could also be thought of as a neuropsychological disconnection, but one where there was impaired access to both perceptual and conceptual stored knowledge, following spared perceptual processing (Figure 6.3).

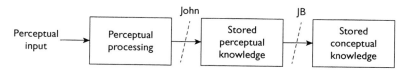

Figure 6.3 A 'disconnection account' of John and patient JB, with the two patients having damage at different stages of access to stored knowledge about objects

However, there were aspects of John's performance that did not fit with this diagnosis. For one thing, John nearly always made visual errors when asked to identify objects – he would name an object as something that had similar features but did not necessarily belong to the same category [58]. For example, he named a spoon as a hammer, a salt cellar as a cotton reel and a line drawing of a nose was called a ladle. It is not clear why visual errors should arise if John had intact perceptual processes but simply failed to access stored perceptual knowledge. Second, John complained that recognition was difficult under particular conditions – for example, when a surface was cluttered with objects or when objects were partially hidden by others (so one object was partially occluded). There seems no reason why making perceptual processing harder by cluttering and occlusion should particularly impair recognition when perceptual processes are intact – John should have perceived the stimuli perfectly well across the different visual conditions. To understand John's problems, we need to explore his perceptual processing in more detail.

Tests of perceptual integration

A first sign that John had a perceptual problem, not a disconnection deficit following normal perception, came from tasks asking him to identify sets of overlapping figures. Irrespective of whether the stimuli were letters or objects, John was substantially worse than age-matched controls at identifying the overlapping shapes [61, 64]. Take the example Figure 6.4, where a camel, a finger and a cannon overlap one another. Even though John could name the individual objects when shown in isolation, he had great difficulty in identifying the same items when they overlapped. A telling reason for this was revealed when, instead of having to name the objects, we required John to copy an exemplar. A set of overlapping shapes was presented above two individual examples (as in Figure 6.4). John was told that one of the bottom examples was in the overlapping drawing and he was asked to draw that exemplar in the overlapping stimulus. He was poor at doing this and often made errors by failing to segment the shapes appropriately, sometimes drawing in parts that belonged to different objects. This indicates that John did indeed have a perceptual problem which is made apparent when there are demands on segmenting contours belonging to different objects.

A further example of John's perceptual difficulties was shown in another copying task where we systematically manipulated the demands on segmentation – from cases where parts of objects did not overlap to cases where complex segmentation processes were required

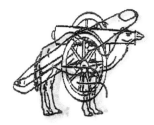

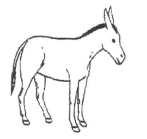 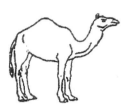

Figure 6.4 Example of a task requiring John to detect and draw the item in the overlapping figures at the top which matches one of the two exemplars shown at the bottom

Source: From Riddoch, M. J., Humphreys, G. W. *et al.* (2008) A tale of two agnosias: distinctions between form and integrative agnosia. *Cognitive Neuropsychology* 25: 56–92, reprinted by permission of the publisher (Taylor & Francis Group, http://www.informaworld.com).

to distinguish one object from another [61]. An example in Figure 6.5 (a) does not require segmentation as there are no overlapping parts. The example in (b) in Figure 6.5 does require segmentation as the 'cross' part of the front shape overlaps the back 'square'. However segmentation here involves coding the occluded (background) shape based on the relations between simple horizontal and vertical edges where the front and back objects overlap. The examples in (c) again require segmentation but they introduce more demands by using oblique edges and having multiple points where segmentation is required. Some of John's drawings are presented alongside the exemplars. While he was good at copying simple shapes not requiring segmentation as in example (a), he made errors as segmentation became more demanding. These errors included drawing in occluded (hidden) edges where they were not present (i.e., John perceptually 'completed' shapes where he should not) and using occlusion to segment apart elements that should have been grouped ('over-segmentation'; see Figure 6.5 (b) (ii)).

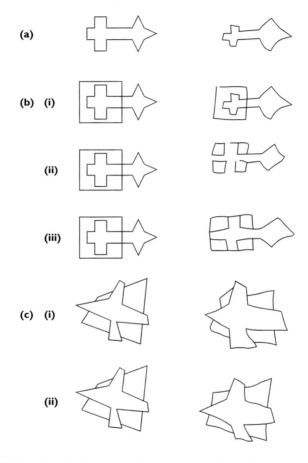

Figure 6.5 Examples of John copying shapes varying in their demands on grouping across occluded edges and segmenting surfaces

Source: From Giersch, A., Humphreys, G. W., Boucart, M. and Koviáks, I. (2000) The computation of occluded contours in visual agnosia: evidence of early computation prior to shape binding and figure-ground coding. *Cognitive Neuropsychology* 17: 731–759, reprinted by permission of the publisher (Taylor & Francis Group, http://www.informaworld.com).

These errors in drawing are intriguing, given John's very good performance when he had simply to group aligned contours without then having to use the groups to construct multi-part objects or to segment between objects (Figure 6.1 above). The results suggest that John was able to carry out elementary forms of grouping between aligned edges; as we noted in Chapter 4, this is a process that may be carried out in early regions of visual cortex (even in area V1). However, John was impaired at a higher stage of perceptual organisation, when multiple shape elements must be formed into parts of more complex shapes – and particularly when there were competing organisations present, such as when one surface sat in front of another. Given the brain lesion suffered by John which affected 'intermediate' visual areas including V2, V3 and V4 (Figure 4.2), then the results suggest that that these intermediate areas construct higher forms of perceptual organisation, where the relations between multiple parts and surfaces of objects are integrated. The stage of processing involving the integration of parts with more holistic representations of surfaces was disrupted. The nature of the disruption may be to introduce 'noise' in the process – this led to both inappropriate grouping (where extra occluded edges were coded where they should not), and inappropriate segmentation (where surfaces were segmented when they should have been grouped to enable a background objects to be coded separately from an object positioned in front).

John's impairments in interlinking grouping and segmentation were also apparent when he had to search and find items – and in everyday life finding something on a cluttered surface gave him enormous difficulties. We assessed this using 'visual search' – a procedure in which the efficiency of finding a target is measured as the number of distractors is varied. We examined John's performance in a variety of search conditions but crucially comparing tasks dependent just on detecting how one feature of the display differs from others (so-called 'feature search') and tasks where the ease of detecting a target depends on grouping between the distractors and segmentation of the target from this group [59, 64]. Examples of the search displays are depicted in Figure 6.6.

In search tasks like this, targets can be detected efficiently if they have a basic feature which differs from distractors (the left panel, where the target has a different overall orientation to the distractors). In this case, the number of distractors present has little effect on target detection – the target 'pops out' and attracts attention. Here, differential activity in early visual regions, selective to contrasting orientations, may lead to the target 'pop out' effect. For normal observers, search is also efficient for targets and distractors such as those shown in the middle panel. In these displays

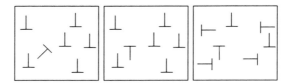

Figure 6.6 Examples of search displays where the target (the T) can be detected either based on a difference in one of its basic features relative to distractors (left panel), the way features combine and can be grouped to segment the target from the distractors (middle panel), or the systematic inspection of each item given (right panel, when targets and distractors have the same basic features and there is not strong grouping across the distractors to produce efficient segmentation of the target.

Source: From Riddoch, M. J. and Humphreys, G. W. (2000). The neuropsychology of object recognition, in Rapp, B. (ed.), *The Handbook of Cognitive Neuropsychology.* Hove: Psychology Press, reprinted by permission of the publisher (Taylor & Francis Group, http://www.informaworld.com).

all the items have the same basic features (all the lines have the same orientation) but targets and distractors have different arrangements of features. In addition, there is a constant feature arrangement across the distractors (so the distractors form a homogeneous group of inverted Ts), and this contrasts with the arrangement of features making the target. Normal participants are able to group the separate homogeneous distractors and then segment them from the target. This rejection of the distractors as a single group enables the target again to 'pop out'. However, search is inefficient for displays such as those shown in the right panel because targets and distractors neither differ in their basic features (as in the left panel), nor do they differ in a consistent arrangement of features across the distractor set. Without the basic feature difference or the possibility of grouping the distractors as a single set distinct from the target, search depends on serial inspection of each item to check if it is the target.

We tested John with displays such as these. We found that he was just as efficient as controls at detecting targets in the basic feature case (left panel) and in the difficult search condition shown in the right panel. This again indicates that John's processing of basic visual features was spared (in the easy feature search), as was his ability to discriminate simple visual elements when processed one at a time (in the difficult case of serial inspection, right panel). However, he was greatly impaired compared with controls when we presented him with the central displays, when controls benefit from the grouping of distractors and the segmentation of the target. This was not for want of practice. We gave John over 3000 trials of practice at the grouping condition, but still he failed to show good target discrimination. There appeared to be a fundamental problem in him grouping complex visual forms to perform efficient segmentation of a display. This provides converging evidence for John having a selective perceptual problem at the level of coding relatively complex groups of forms.

In addition to demonstrating that John was abnormally affected by overlap, occlusion and grouping, we also found that his object recognition was abnormally affected by the speed of presenting stimuli [58]. For instance, if we reduce the exposure duration of an object for normal participants from 1 second to just a tenth of that (100 ms), there are only small effects on our ability to identify the object – it remains quite easy to identify objects shown only for this brief duration. However this was not the case for John. For items he was able to identify with long exposures, he was strikingly impaired as the exposure duration decreased. The limits on John's poor integration of parts of complex objects were exaggerated under the reduced exposure conditions.

Some conclusions

Taken together, the results indicate that John was not in fact an associative agnosic, in the sense as set out by Lissauer, but he suffered a form of apperceptive agnosia in that there was a fundamental underlying perceptual impairment. The problem was not at the stage of coding the primitive elements of form, nor even in grouping those elements into simple two-dimensional shapes. Rather, the problem was at a stage of higher-level grouping and segmentation of parts and surfaces of objects. This in turn indicates that the apperceptive-associative distinction put forward by Lissauer in 1890 is too simplistic to capture the full range of disturbances that can affect human visual perception – with some perceptual processes being impaired in John's case but others being spared. We proposed that patients such as John suffer from a distinct form of agnosia, which we termed *integrative agnosia*, to reflect (1) the critical problem in grouping and segmentation of complex elements, and (2) that this is a distinct category of problem, separate from both form agnosia (indexed by performance on the 'Efron' task) and associative agnosia (where perceptual processing is intact, in a case such as patient JB; Chapter 5). Patients with integrative agnosia have a perceptual deficit that is higher level than the problem apparent in patients who fail the basic Efron test but they still do not suffer a purely associative problem.

Chapter 7

Seeing the whole

> It's as if I see things slightly out of focus, not to my eyes, if you understand, but to my brain . . .
>
> (John)

Although patients such as John are poor at integrating parts into organised representations of objects and although they can over-segment cluttered, complex images, there is a paradox. John, for example, never seemed to be unaware of all the elements present in a scene, though he might organise them inappropriately in his perception. This contrasts with patients with another visual disorder known as simultanagnosia, which occurs after damage to more dorsal parts of the cortical visual stream (affecting the pathway from the occipital to the parietal cortex). Simultanagnosic patients can show a lack of awareness about all of the elements in a scene, only reporting the presence of a single object at a time. Simultanagnosics can also produce naming errors of a type that John never made, which was to name a part of an object as if it is the whole object, while showing no awareness that there are other parts present. An example might be naming a bicycle as a wheel [65]. John might make segmentation errors in which he assigned overlapping parts to the wrong objects, but he always reported that there were other stimuli present on such occasions. He might misidentify a pushbike as a motorbike or even as part of a watermill, but he would always notice the elements that comprised the frame and handles of the bike. This suggests that agnosic patients such as John do have some holistic information about objects, even if it appears insufficient to identify the object or even to constrain how the parts of objects are integrated.

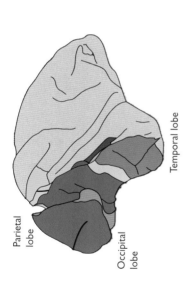

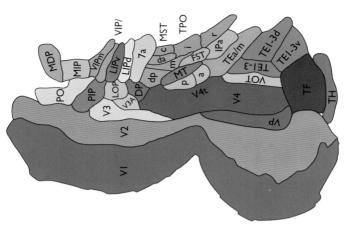

Parietal lobe

Occipital lobe

Temporal lobe

Figure 4.2 See p. 25. Some of the different visual areas in the monkey brain revealed through single cell electrode recording. On the left is a figure of the monkey right hemisphere (the purple region is at the back of the brain). On the right, the brain is laid out on a flat surface to reveal the different regions more clearly than when they are shown on the very convoluted surface of the real brain. V1 corresponds to the primary visual cortex, which receives signals from the eye. The remaining areas, shown in different colours here for illustrative purposes, are defined by the properties of the cells there (see the text for details).

Source: Modified from Van Essen, D. C., Lewis, J. W., Drury, H. A., Hadjikhani, N., Tootell, R. B. H., Bakircioglu, M. and Miller, M. I. (2001) Mapping visual cortex in monkeys and humans using surface-based atlases. *Vision Research* 41: 1359–1378, with permission from Elsevier.

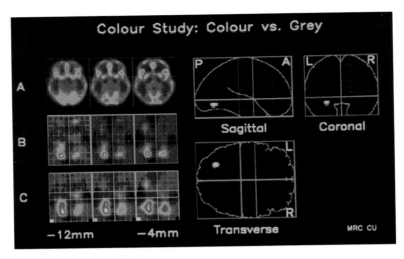

Figure 4.3 See p. 26. A 'subtraction' image showing brain regions more strongly activated by a colour Mondrian than by a grey-level image matched to the Mondrian for brightness, revealed by PET imaging. The images on the left are colour-coded to illustrate regions that showed greater activity for coloured over grey-level stimuli. These are horizontal (transverse) slices of the brain, with the back of the brain shown at the bottom of each slice. The figures on the right are outlines of the brain shown from different views – looking side-on (sagittal; back of the brain on the left), looking at a vertical slice (coronal) and looking at a horizontal slice (transverse; back of the brain on the left of the figure). The highlighted region marked on the outline in the transverse slice falls towards the back of the left hemisphere but significant activation can be found too in the equivalent area in the right hemisphere (shown by the 'hotspots' on both sides of the brain in part C of the figure).

Source: Republished with permission of The Society of Neuroscience, from Zeki, S. *et al.* (1991) A direct demonstration of functional specialisation in human visual cortex. *Journal of Neuroscience* 11: 641–649, permission conveyed through Copyright Clearance Centre, Inc.

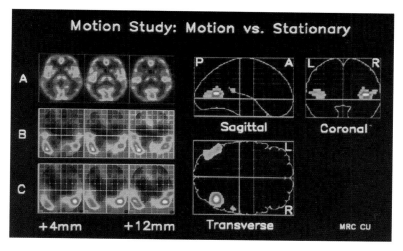

Figure 4.4 See p. 26. A 'subtraction' image from the PET study of Zeki and colleagues (1991) showing brain regions more strongly activated by moving relative to stationary dots (in the transverse slices on the left, brain regions are colour-coded to illustrate their level of activity – 'hot' colours depict areas with more activity). The outline brains on the right indicate the active regions that define area MT. Note that these regions fall higher in the brain (at more superior locations) and they are more lateral than the colour regions shown in Figure 4.3).

Source: Republished with permission of The Society of Neuroscience, from Zeki, S. *et al.* (1991) A direct demonstration of functional specialisation in human visual cortex. *Journal of Neuroscience* 11: 641–649, permission conveyed through Copyright Clearance Centre, Inc.

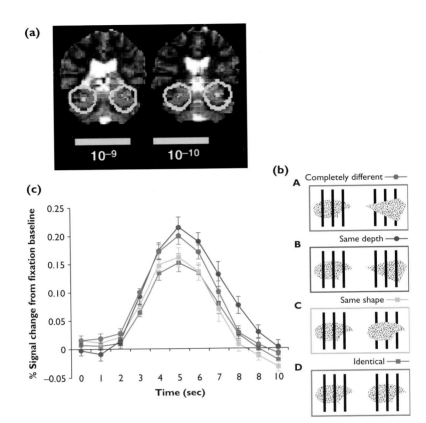

Figure 4.10 (a) Activity in the LOC within the ventral visual stream. (b) Stimuli used to probe activity in the LOC. Pairs of stimuli would be different shapes at different depth, different shapes at the same depth, the same shape but appearing at different depths, behind or in front of the bars, or identical shapes both in front of or behind the bars. (c) The profile of LOC activity over time to the second stimulus. There is reduced activity (adaptation) for the second stimulus when it is the same shape irrespective of whether it is at the same depth, occluded then not occluded.

Source: From Kourtzi, Z. and Kanwisher, N. (2001) Representation of perceived object shape by the human lateral occipital complex. *Science* 293: 1506–1509. Reprinted with permission from AAAS.

Object Processing

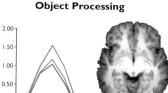

Background Scene Processing

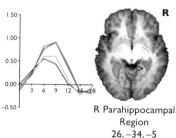

R

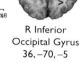

R Inferior
Occipital Gyrus
36, –70, –5

R Parahippocampal
Region
26, –34, –5

Figure 4.11 Illustration of object- and scene-level visual adaptation. The graphs show a measure of oxygenation levels in the blood in particular brain regions (the Blood Oxygenation Level Dependent, or BOLD, response, recorded using fMRI). Since brain regions more actively engaged in a task consume more oxygen, the BOLD response is typically taken as a proxy index of neuronal activity. In the present case the BOLD response is shown in each graph for several conditions: when objects were repeated in the same and different scenes (blue and green curves), when scenes were repeated with different objects (orange curves) and trials where both the objects and the scenes differed (red curves). The left figure indicates that there was reduced activation bilaterally (in both the left and right hemispheres) in the inferior occipital gyrus when objects repeated, compared with when they differed – shown in the horizontal (transverse) brain slice (top = the front of the brain). Note that there was overlap of the red and orange-labelled BOLD responses for the conditions when the objects changed, and these conditions showed increased activity compared with the blue and green-labelled responses when the objects were re-presented. Right: Illustration of scene-level adaptation in the right parahippocampal gyrus. In this case, brain activity was reduced when scenes were repeated with either the same or different objects (blue and orange curves) compared with when the scenes changes and either the objects remained the same or they changed too (green and red curves, which overlapped in this case). The transverse brain slice shows the differences between the scene repeat and scene-change trials which was significant in the left and right parahippocampal regions.

Source: Republished with permission of The Society of Neuroscience, from Goh, J. O. S. *et al.* (2004) Cortical areas involved in object, background, and object background processing revealed with functional magnetic resonance adaptation. *Journal of Neuroscience* 24: 10223–10228, permission conveyed through Copyright Clearance Centre, Inc.

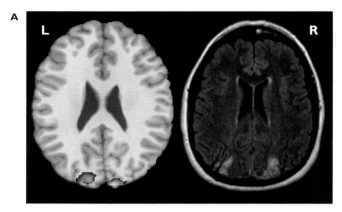

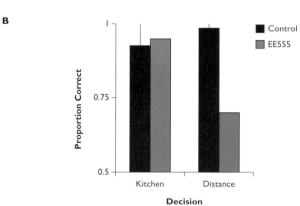

Figure 4.13 Top left: brain areas showing adaptation (reduced activation) in normal observers when objects were repeated at the same depth compared with when they appeared at different depths. Top right: regions damaged inpatient EE5555 (marked by the red circles). Bottom: the proportion of correct responses made by control participants and patient EE555 when required either to judge whether objects belonged in the kitchen or their relative depth. The patient was selectively impaired at judging depth, despite being able to recognize whether the objects belonged in the kitchen.

Source: From Berryhill, M. E. and Olson, I. R. (2009) The representation of object distance: evidence from neuroimaging and neuropsychology. *Frontiers in Human Neuroscience* 3(43).

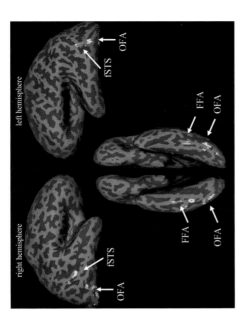

Grasping > Reaching

Intact > Scrambled Objects

L   R

z = 48   z = -7

Figure 4.14 See p. 38. Left: brain regions showing greater activity when a grasping rather than a pointing action had to be made. Right: brain regions more active when intact rather than scrambled images of objects were presented. In the latter case, the activated regions conform to the Lateral Occipital Complex (LOC). The regions affected by grasping are more superior in the brain (in parietal cortex) than the regions responding to intact objects. This is indicated by the difference in the z values shown in each slide, which represents the height at which the transverse scan was taken. The higher the z value, the more superior or dorsal the scan.

Source: Culham, J. C. et al. (2003) Visually guided grasping produces fMRI activation in dorsal but not ventral stream brain areas. *Experimental Brain Research* 153: 180–189. Reproduced with kind permission from Springer Science + Business Media.

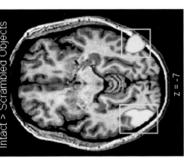

left hemisphere

OFA

fSTS

FFA

OFA

right hemisphere

fSTS

OFA

FFA

OFA

Figure 4.17 Brain areas selectively activated by faces relative to other stimuli. Faces particularly activate a region in the occipital cortex (the occipital face area, OFA), the fusiform gyrus (the fusiform face area, FFA) and the superior temporal sulcus (fSTS).

Source: From Kanwisher, N. and Yovel, G. (2006) The fusiform face area: a cortical region specialised for the perception of faces. *Philosophical Transactions of the Royal Society, Series B* 361: 2109–2128, by permission of the Royal Society.

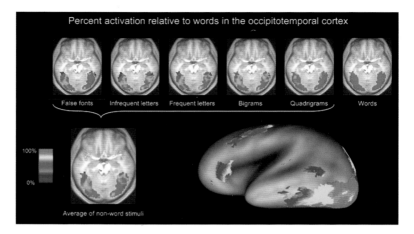

Average of non-word stimuli

Figure 4.20 Percentage of activation, relative to words, for different types of symbols. There is less activation of more anterior regions of the left fusiform gyrus as the symbols become less word-like (coloured to indicate decreasing overlap of activity with words).

Source: Reprinted from Vinckier, F. *et al.* (2007). Hierarchical coding of letter strings in the ventral stream: dissecting the inner organization of the visual word-form system. *Neuron* 55: 143–156, with permission from Elsevier.

Figure 9.1 See p. 91. Example stimuli used to assess residual colour processing in John. Each display consisted of elements shown in one quadrant here, with a white line dividing the top and bottom halves of each display. On consecutive displays John was presented with either the top pair of stimuli shown here or the bottom pair. In the top pair, the first stimulus [left] has contrasting patches differing in colour, while the second stimulus does not. In the bottom pair, the first stimulus has contrasting patches differing in brightness, while the second stimulus does not. In each case, the task was to decide whether the first or the second stimulus had differing patches.

Source: Reprinted from Troscianko, T. *et al.* (1996). Human colour discrimination based on a non-parvocellular pathway. *Current Biology* 6: 200–210, with permission from Elsevier.

Processing silhouettes

We tried to put this supposition to the test. We examined John's ability to match shapes under conditions of overlap and occlusion, comparing his performance with overlapping and occluded items to a baseline condition where the same shapes were present but separated (not over-lapping/occluded) (Figure 7.1) [61]. Perhaps not surprisingly, given our previous results, we found that John was relatively good at making the matches with separated shapes but he was impaired with overlapping and occluded stimuli. The interesting condition was when he was presented with silhouettes of the items, when his performance improved, relative to the overlapping and occluded conditions. It is not that silhouettes are generally easier, since the control participants performed at the same level as with overlapping and occluded stimuli. To explain these results, we suggested that John was able to respond to the silhouettes in a rela-tively holistic way, with each triplet coded as a global shape. This may be less possible with unfilled shapes, which have strong edge cues which may automatically recruit segmentation processes and a more parts-based processing strategy.

We were able to confirm the improved performance for silhouettes in a range of other tasks where we assessed access to stored knowledge and not just shape processing. For example, he was better at identifying silhouettes than line drawings of the same items and, again relative to when he was presented with line drawings, he was better at object deci-sions when the objects and nonobjects appeared as silhouettes [58, 66]. We propose that the lack of internal detail in silhouettes gave rise to a perceptual advantage because they were less likely than line drawings to be over-segmented on the basis of internal edges.

Hierarchical stimuli

The argument for John being able to compute some global properties of stimuli is given strongest support from studies using local-global hier-archical shapes (see Chapter 4 Figure 4.8). We have noted that, when given hierarchical global letters made out of independent local letters, normal participants can show a 'global precedence effect' – they can be faster to respond to global than local targets, and their responses to local targets can be disrupted if the global form has a conflicting identity. This global precedence effect may depend on observers encoding a coarse (low-spatial frequency) representation of the global form. If this coarse representation is sufficiently distinctive, then it can serve for object rec-ognition. However, with many objects (and especially those with similar

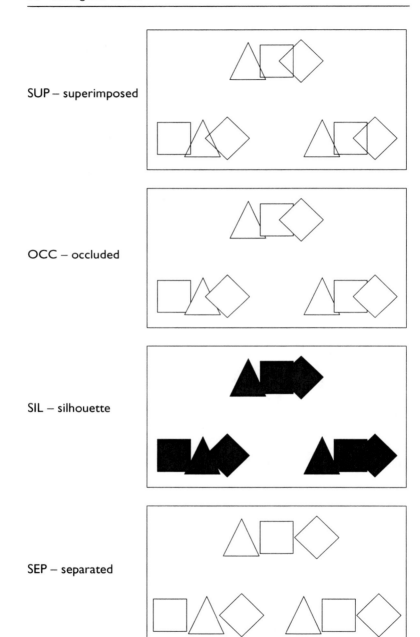

SUP – superimposed

OCC – occluded

SIL – silhouette

SEP – separated

Figure 7.1 (opposite) Shape matching stimuli used with John. The task was to judge which of the two lower sets of shapes matched the upper shapes. The stimuli could have the same shapes present but in different spatial orders. The conditions were as follows: in SUP the shapes were superimposed line drawings. In OCC the stimuli were occluding line drawings. In SIL the items were silhouettes of the shapes but without internal dividing lines. In SEP, the stimuli were spatially separated line drawings.

Source: From Giersch, A., Humphreys, G. W., Boucart, M. and Kovíáks, I. (2000) The computation of occluded contours in visual agnosia: evidence of early computation prior to shape binding and figure-ground coding. *Cognitive Neuropsychology* 17: 731–759, reprinted by permission of the publisher (Taylor & Francis Group, http://www.informaworld.com).

global structures) a coarse global representation will not be distinctive enough to enable recognition to occur, and recognition may then be dependent on a parts-based approach. Consistent with this last argument, we noted that John was better at identifying non-living than living things, and this may reflect the similar global structures of many living things which limits the use of coarse global structures for recognition. Indeed, presenting stimuli as silhouettes was more helpful for non-living things (the scissors in Figure 7.2) than living things (the camel), presumably because the coarse visual information better differentiated between non-living things and also stopped non-living things from being segmented inappropriately into independent parts [64].

These ideas were explored in studies of hierarchical object recognition in John [64, 65]. We presented local-global letter stimuli such as those shown in Figure 7.3 and John (and control participants) had to identify either the local or the global forms. Somewhat to our surprise we found that John showed a large global precedence effect – stronger even than that found in the control subjects. This global precedence effect was

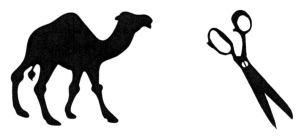

Figure 7.2 Example silhouettes of living and non-living objects

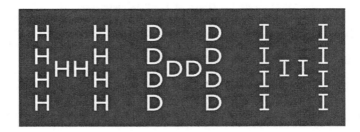

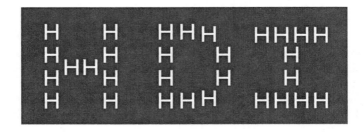

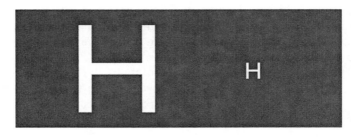

Figure 7.3 Example hierarchical stimuli. The task required John to identify whether the global shape was an H or a D (stimuli in the top row, all Hs), or whether the local letter was an H or D (stimuli in the middle row, all Hs again). There were also 'baseline' stimuli, matched to the size of either the global (bottom row, left) or local shape (bottom row, right).

due in part to his responses being very slow to local elements embedded within the more global shapes – indeed his responses to these local shapes were much slower when they fell within the global forms compared with when they were the same size but appeared in isolation (in a baseline condition). It cannot be argued that these local shapes were simply too small to be resolved.

How do we reconcile the finding that John can respond to the global shape of hierarchical letters with our other evidence that he is impaired at perceptual integration of parts into more complex perceptual representations? In Chapter 4 we argued that the global shape of a stimulus can be conveyed by low spatial frequency information, which provides the coarse overall shape of a stimulus. There is evidence of separate cell types in early visual cortex, 'parvocellular' and 'magnocellular' cells, which respond selectively to high and low spatial frequency components in an image [68]. John's fast responses to global forms may be based on the rapid-acting magnocellular cells, which can respond to the coarse outline of the shape. While this may support the identification of simple letter stimuli, it is insufficient to support the recognition of more complex shapes, where a parts-based analysis is needed to enhance the coarse visual description. As we argued in Chapter 6, it is this parts-based analysis that is impaired in John.

The argument that the coarse coding of shape is preserved enables us to account for the results with silhouettes, where he performed relatively well. Silhouettes may be identified from their coarse global forms, and do not depend on the further elaboration by local parts (which can be obscured). John's worse performance with line drawings, compared with silhouettes, suggests that the 'noise' introduced by his impaired parts-based analysis disrupts the low spatial frequency representation that might otherwise be available. It is not simply that John's low spatial frequency representation is not elaborated by a parts-based analysis, but that the parts-based analysis was disruptive to the coarse shape coding.

The contrast between poor parts-based recognition and the ability to code coarse global structure was also shown using matching tasks, where John simply had to decide if two stimuli were the same or different [69]. He was presented with stimuli such as those shown in Figure 7.4. The task was to judge if two images were identical or mirror-reflected. The images were either line drawings or fragmented forms which were either easy or hard for normal participants to identify ('well' or 'poorly' structured forms). Also, when the shapes were mirror-reflected, they either had the same overall orientation (top items) or they had a different overall orientation (bottom items). Unlike normal participants, John showed no advantage for well-structured over poorly structured fragmented forms, suggesting that he was insensitive to the ease of coding the parts into whole forms. At the same time, John was considerably better at judging that the stimuli differed when their overall orientation changed (bottom items) than when they were mirror-reflected but had the same overall orientation (top items). He was sensitive to the coarse global orientation but not to the finer-grained difference between well-structured and poorly-structured parts.

We tested whether the coarse global information that John appeared able to encode could activate his stored knowledge to at least some degree, even if he was unable to fully identify the stimulus. To do this we had him carry out a 'global shape' matching task. He was presented with three figures such as those depicted in Figure 7.5 and he had to decide which of the two lower stimuli had the same global shape as the upper

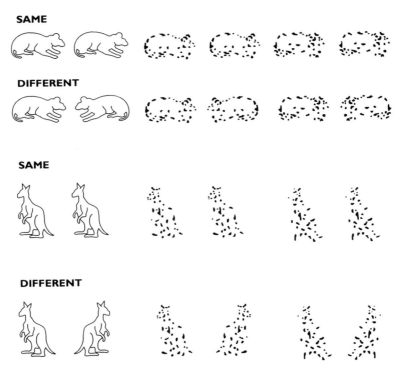

Figure 7.4 Pairs of stimuli used by Boucart and Humphreys (1992) in a study of shape matching. The task was to decide if pairs of images were the same or mirror-reflected ('different'). On different trials the images could have the same overall orientation or they could differ in overall orientation.

Source: Reprinted from Boucart, M. and Humphreys, G. W. (1992) The computation of perceptual structure from collinearity and closure: normality and pathology. *Neuropsychologia* 30: 527–546, with permission from Elsevier.

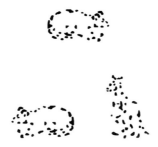

Figure 7.5 Stimuli from a 'global shape' matching test, where the task was to decide which of the lower figures had the same global shape as the upper figure. Normal participants are slowed in these judgements when the distractor (lower right) belongs to the same category as the target object (lower left). In contrast, John showed no effect of whether the objects belonged to the same category.

Source: Reprinted from Boucart, M. and Humphreys, G. W. (1992) The computation of perceptual structure from collinearity and closure: normality and pathology. *Neuropsychologia* 30: 527–546, with permission from Elsevier.

stimulus. When normal participants perform this task, their responses are slowed if the distractor item belongs to the same category as the target – we cannot help but register the category of the stimuli, and similarity at the category level makes it difficult to reject the distractor as being perceptually different. John, however, showed no effect of category similarity though he was able to match items based on their global shape. There was no evidence of him accessing stored knowledge about objects from their global shape [70]. With normal participants, access to stored knowledge seems to depend on the rapid integration of the local parts – a process deficient in John.

Brain mechanisms

We were also able to test the brain mechanisms mediating John's responses to local and global stimuli, and this helps to throw light on the way in which he perceived complex forms. To do this, we used fMRI, which measures blood oxygen levels in different brain regions when people perform tasks. We scanned John while he responded to local and global letters and contrasted the effects with those present in another agnosic patient, Sue, whom we were also fortunate to work with. Sue's case differs from that of John in an interesting manner, since she had suffered more 'dorsal' brain lesions (affecting the occipito-parietal rather

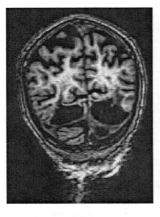
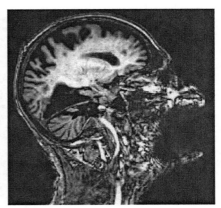
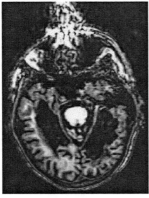

Figure 7.6 Left: structural MRI scan for John. Right: structural MRI scan for Sue. Note that Sue's lesions were more dorsal (higher in the brain) and more posterior (to the back of the brain) compared with John.

Source: From Riddoch, M. J., Humphreys, G. W., Akhtar, N., Allen, H., Bracewell, R. M. and Schofield, A. J. (2008). A tale of two agnosias: distinctions between form and integrative agnosia. *Cognitive Neuropsychology* 25: 56–92, reprinted by permission of the publisher (Taylor & Francis Group, http://www. informaworld.com).

than the occipito-temporal cortex) – so there were complementary changes in ventral (John) and dorsal (Sue) occipital cortex in the two cases (see Figure 7.6) [64, 71].

Sue also presented with an opposite pattern of performance to John, when required to identify local and global forms – whereas John showed

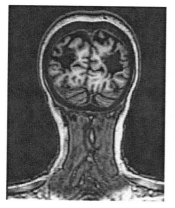
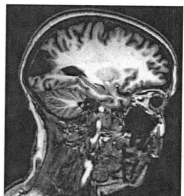
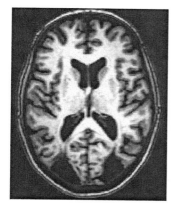

Figure 7.6 continued.

strong global precedence, Sue had strong local precedence and found it difficult to identify the global forms. This suggests that the more dorsal lesions sustained by Sue are involved in coding global forms. In contrast, the more ventral areas damaged in John are involved in the perception of local shape, and so disrupt the identification of local more than global shapes.

To evaluate John's response to hierarchical shapes, we analysed activation in the brain regions lesioned in Sue, but which were spared in John [64]. We also conducted the reverse analyses – examining the activity in Sue's brain in the regions that were lesioned in John, but intact in her. The results are presented in Figure 7.7, for John, Sue and age-matched control participants. The regions listed for the controls represent the dorsal areas lesioned in Sue and the ventral areas lesioned in John. Relative

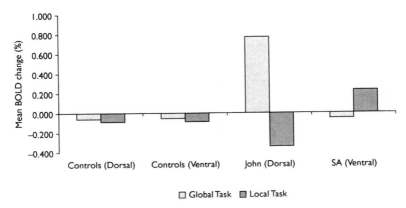

Figure 7.7 Brain activity for normal control participants, John and SA when responding to global and local shapes (making up a hierarchical form; see Figure 7.5). Relative to the controls, John shows a much stronger response to global shape within the dorsal area of cortex lesioned in SA. In contrast, SA shows a much stronger response to local shape in the ventral area of cortex damaged in John. The data suggest that the dorsal cortex is recruited when global shapes are identified and ventral cortex when local shapes are identified.

to the activation shown by the controls in these regions, the results from the two agnosic patients are striking. John had massively increased activity in the dorsal region when the task was to identify the global shape. Sue, in contrast, had a greatly increased response in the ventral region when she had to identify local shapes. Thus each agnosic patient had a greater than usual response within the preserved brain region responding to a particular property of the stimuli – the global shape (in dorsal occipital cortex, in John), and the local elements (in ventral occipital cortex, in Sue).

It is interesting to review the implications of this for the way we might normally process hierarchical figures. The increased responses in the patients suggest that, in normal subjects, there are interactions between the processing of local and global properties of stimuli – with activation in one area modulating the other. For example, there may be less strong activity in the dorsal area responding to global shape when there is concurrent high activation in the ventral region responding to local shape. John, missing this ventral modulation due to his brain lesion, shows an increased dorsal response to global shape. The opposite holds for Sue. Her lesion affects the dorsal processing of global shape and thus prevents this from modulating activity that is driven by the local shape in her spared ventral cortex. John sees the global shape of an object even more strongly than controls and Sue sees the local shape even more strongly than the controls. In John's case, however, this global information is undifferentiated and not supplemented by a parts-based analysis. As a consequence object recognition is limited, as we observed.

Conclusion

Our analysis with John indicated that he responded strongly to the global shape of objects, so that he showed an abnormally large advantage in responding to the global form relative to the local parts of objects. This was associated with exaggerated neural activation in the brain region responding to global shape (in the dorsal occipital cortex). The results indicate that the brain regions responding to local and global forms normally interact. Lesioning one region changes the response in the other. In Chapter 6 we presented data demonstrating that John was impaired at parts-based analysis of complex stimuli. It follows that his strong global response here is not derived from a parts-based analysis but from independent coding of coarse global structure.

Chapter 8

What's in a face?

Lately I have been trying to go by the eyebrows but this has not proved successful.

(John)

Face recognition

In Chapter 5 we reviewed evidence that face recognition may operate in a relatively 'modular' fashion, independent of the visual processes supporting the recognition of other objects. Some of the strongest arguments for the 'modularity' of face recognition comes from patients who have selective difficulty in identifying faces but who do not have difficulties with objects – the disorder labelled 'prosopagnosia'. We have worked with one patient with a very 'pure' prosopagnosia, FB [72]. FB was formerly a shop detective who depended on good face recognition abilities for her livelihood. However, due to an arteriovenus malformation, FB suffered a brain lesion in the area of the fusiform gyrus in her right hemisphere. Following this, she had severe difficulties in recognising faces – even those of close family members. This appeared to be a problem in perception rather than her memory, since she was poor at making perceptual judgements about whether pairs of faces were the same or not, especially if they were depicted in slightly different views – that is, she was impaired at tests where long-term memory for known faces was not required. For example, FB fell below the level expected from normal controls on the test depicted in Figure 8.1. In contrast to her impaired perception of faces, FB was strikingly good at object identification. An illustration of this is that she was able to name objects such as those presented in Figure 8.2 to at least the level of accuracy found in university students, whom we tested as controls – correctly calling the animal a 'wildebeest' and the object a 'Tantalus'. We failed to find any problem with object recognition despite her face recognition impairments. Findings from patients such as FB are consistent with the view that the brain has developed at least some specialist processes that are necessary for face recognition but not for recognising other types of objects.

Unlike FB, John was impaired at recognising many different objects, so the problems he had with faces were not selective. Nevertheless they were dramatic. As a British subject in the 1980s, it was striking that John was steadfastly unable to recognise Margaret Thatcher, whose image was

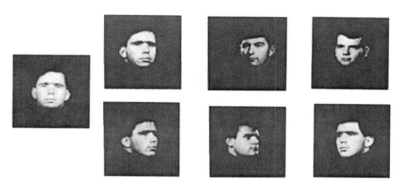

Figure 8.1 The 'Benton' face matching test requires the participant to judge which of the six faces on the right match the face on the left (answer, there are three!). Performance is taken as an index of face perception.

Source: From Benton, A. L. *et al.* (1994) *Contributions to Neuropsychological Assessment.* New York: Oxford University Press. By permission of Oxford University Press, USA.

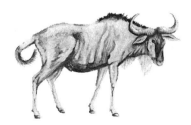
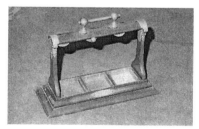

Figure 8.2 The object naming task of McKenna and Warrington (1997).

Source: From McKenna, P. and Warrington, E. (1997) *Category Specific Names Test.* Hove: Psychology Press, reprinted by permission of the publisher (Taylor & Francis Group, http://www.informaworld.com).

very pervasive at the time. Given a photograph of someone, he was not only poor at knowing who the person was, he was barely above chance at judging their gender, age or facial emotion. Like FB, the problem appeared to be perceptual in nature, and John failed completely at matching faces across different views (see Figure 8.1). This was not a general problem in 'person recognition', however. For example, John was perfectly able to recognise an individual from his or her voice and he reported trying to identify his wife from her gait when she walked. This contrast was brought home to us when we once called unexpectedly at his house and, on answering the door, John gave absolutely no sign of realising who we were – despite the fact that we had known each other for over three years by this stage. However when we spoke, recognition was immediate.

We attempted to assess which particular aspects of face processing were impaired. We gave John a matching task in which he had to decide whether consecutive images were the same or different faces, using the stimuli introduced by Takane and Sergent which we discussed in Chapter 4 (Figure 4.16) [31]. We measured the time it took John to detect changes between faces which differed in just one (e.g., the eyes), two (e.g., eyes and chin) or three features (eyes, chin and hairstyle). Whereas normal observers become faster at discriminating faces when they differed in more features, John showed no added benefit when more feature differences were added. For example, his fastest responses were when the faces differed just in their chins, not when there were contrasts in the chin, eyes and hairline too (for faces differing in their chins his response time was 1.25 sec.; when the faces differed in their chins, eyes and hairline, his mean response time was 1.32 sec.). The normal benefit from making the faces vary in more features can be attributed to observers responding to configural changes in the relations between facial features [31]. John did not benefit from these configural changes.

We tested this further using stimuli such as those shown in Figure 8.3. The task with these stimuli was to decide whether the internal features of the faces – their eyes and mouth – were in their normal (upright) orientation or whether they were inverted. When a full face was present and the internal features were inverted, then the orientations of the internal and external features of the faces opposed one another – the manipulation of 'Thatcherisation' (which we introduced in Chapter 4; see Figure 4.15) [73]. Normal observers responded efficiently to faces that were normal, upright and whole (top left panel), and responses to these 'whole' stimuli were at least as fast as to when the parts were present alone – even though the whole faces are visually more complex.

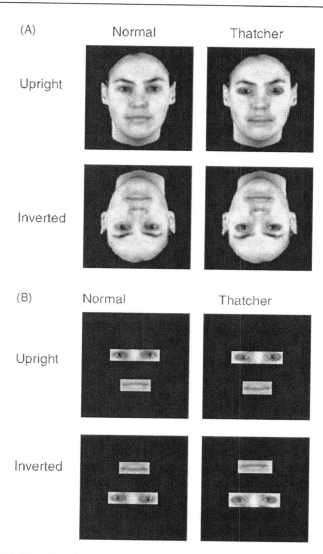

Figure 8.3 Example of normal and Thatcherised faces used by Boutsen and Humphreys (2002). With both whole faces and face parts, the task was to decide if the internal features (the eyes and mouth) were the correct way up or inverted.

Source: Reprinted from Boutsen, L. and Humphreys, G. W. (2002). Face context interferes with local part processing in a prosopagnosic patient. *Neuropsychologia* 40: 2305–2313.

John showed a quite different pattern of performance to the 'norm'. He was much better at deciding whether the face features were inverted when he received the 'parts' compared with when he was presented with the whole face. Also, he tended to perform better when the whole face was turned upside down compared to when it was upright (bottom left images vs. top left images in Figure 8.3). Again these results indicate that John was not helped by the configuration of features present in whole, upright faces – indeed the presence of the whole face disrupted his ability to discriminate the parts. The tendency to perform better with inverted than upright faces is also interesting. How can John be worse with upright faces when normal observers are so much better? This reversed effect suggests that John did process the configural information in upright faces, but instead of helping him, this information hindered his perception. This can be explained if John computes a 'noisy' configuration of features from the upright face, which then impairs his perception. However, if the saliency of the configuration is reduced by turning the face upside down, then the disruption from the faulty configural representation is reduced and performance improves. This counter-intuitive better performance on inverted rather than upright faces has been noted previously in some prosopagnosic patients [74]. We are reminded here of John's increased identification of silhouettes relative to line drawings, which we reported in Chapter 7. Both here when he was presented with faces, and earlier when he was presented with line drawings, the availability of a richer representation (of the upright facial configuration or the line drawing) impairs rather than aids his performance.

Judging emotion and using biological motion

John's perceptual problems in processing faces not only affected his ability to recognise people, but it also disrupted his ability to judge an individual's emotional state from their face. Like face recognition, judgements of emotion are affected by the configuration of features in a face. This is shown in studies using stimuli such as those depicted in Figure 8.4, where the top and bottom halves of faces convey different emotions (angry eyes, happy mouth). When asked to decide if the top half of the face is angry or happy, normal observers are faster to make judgements when the two half faces are separated (left, Figure 8.4) compared with when they are placed together to form a new 'face composite' (right, Figure 8.4). With the new composite, it is difficult to attend to just a part of the face without also processing information about the other parts of the 'whole' (here conveying a different emotion) [75].

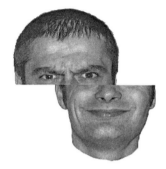 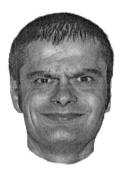

Figure 8.4 Example faces with conflicting emotions (top face = angry, bottom face = happy). Normal observers are faster to judge the emotion of one half when the faces are separated (left) compared with when they form a new composite (right).

Source: Reprinted from Baudouin, J.-Y. and Humphreys, G. W. (2006). Compensatory strategies in processing facial emotions: evidence from prosopagnosia. *Neuropsychologia* 44: 1361–1369, with permission from Elsevier.

Relative to normal observers, John was impaired at judging facial emotions. For example, with the images illustrated in Figure 8.4, he made 16 per cent errors when categorising one half of the face as angry or happy; in contrast, normal observers were faultless (though slowed in the composite condition). Moreover there was a *qualitative* difference in John's performance, since he was unaffected by whether the faces were separated or composite. He was insensitive to the configuration of features in the composite image – just as he was insensitive to facial configurations when matching faces. These problems were also not confined to judging emotion but were also found when John was asked to determine someone's gender – at least when the face was denuded of obvious signs (long hair, 5 o'clock shadow, obvious make-up) [75].

Although John was poor at judging facial emotion and gender when he was presented with static images, he conveyed no sign of this in everyday life. When placed in a social situation John seemed able to judge the emotions and genders of the people present. Of course, emotions can be registered using different kinds of information – from a person's voice or their body language – and John was sensitive to these non-facial cues. But, in addition to this, facial emotion in real life can be conveyed by patterns of movement – as a person smiles or frowns. We evaluated if John could detect emotion from patterns of movement, despite his deficit with static images. To isolate movement, we used 'moving light point' displays [76]. To create such a display, human models had luminous dots painted on their faces and a video was taken of each face in the dark. When the individual stays still, all that can be seen is a pattern of dots. However, when the individual smiles or frowns, the emotion is conveyed immediately by the way the luminous dots move – we can respond to the motion signals in order to discriminate the emotion. When shown light point displays of different emotions, John was able to discriminate the facial emotion at the same level as controls. He also performed at a control level in judging the gender of the face [76]. The results indicate that John could use motion information to form emotion and gender judgements, despite his dramatic impairments in using static cues from faces. The findings fit with the idea we presented in Chapter 4, that different brain regions support the coding of static form and motion form faces and John had a problem with static but not motion information. The results are also consistent with evidence from brain imaging results in normal participants showing that brain regions responding to facial motion (the superior temporal sulcus) are separate from those responding to facial identity (e.g., the fusiform gyrus) [33]. It has been argued that common forms of 'biological motion', such as moving faces, are processed via specialised brain regions sensitive to these ecologically important signals. These brain regions were spared in John's case.

Although John could use pattern of facial motion to judge gender and emotion, he was less adept at using motion when making judgements about a person's identity [77]. We presented John with images of static and moving faces. In one case there were faces of either famous or unknown people and the task was to decide whether the person was familiar or unfamiliar. In a second case only familiar faces were used and John had to associate a name with each face. In these tasks, both of which required John to code the identity of the face, John was not helped by facial motion and he performed poorly relative to controls. For example, for both moving and static faces he was no better than chance at discriminating whether the faces were of familiar or unfamiliar people – a task that control participants found trivially easy. On the other hand when he was simply asked to judge whether two images showed the same person, he performed better with moving than static faces. In this last study, different movement patterns were used when the images depicted the same person, so John was not simply matching the faces on the basis of how they moved. We conclude instead that John was able to use the motion information to derive a representation of facial structure sufficient to discriminate one individual from another. Nevertheless, this representation remained of little use for judging the familiarity of the face (as he was impaired with moving and static faces alike).

We can think of these results in various ways. One possibility is that John was reliant on the 'biological motion' system, in the superior temporal sulcus, but this system only computes relatively coarse representations and not the kind of configural cues that may be needed to identify an individual. It can be used to tell apart two clearly different faces, but not exactly who each person is. A second possibility is that this biological motion system can compute configural information, but John has a problem in matching this information with his memory. To evaluate this, we tested John's memory for faces.

Memory for faces

Good face recognition depends on being able to match the representations being computed from the stimulus with our memories of an individual. This can be illustrated by the not uncommon experience of failing to recognise someone we have not seen for a period if their appearance has changed in the meantime – such failures reflect a mismatch between the information we code from the individual and our outdated memory of what they look like. We tested John's memory for faces by having him report on the features of individuals he knew before his stroke [78]. For example, we asked him questions such as:

Was Winston Churchill bald or not?
Does Eric Morcambe[1] wear glasses?

John did well on these tests, performing as well as control participants. However, we can note that these questions just required John to remember one salient feature about the person – it did not rely on the kinds of information that might be used when we visually recognise someone – notably the configuration of facial features. To evaluate John's memory for configural information, we asked him to judge which two of three named individuals looked more alike. For example:

Who looks more like Elizabeth Taylor? Joan Collins or Barbara Windsor?[2]

Now, unlike his good performance when quizzed about single features of faces, John was impaired when his performance was compared with that of controls. It appeared that his memory specifically for the configural properties of faces was disrupted. Again various interpretations of this are possible. One is that John's brain lesion has disrupted his long-term memory for face configurations – and this can limit face recognition whether the visual input is static or moving (see above). A somewhat different idea is that, when we remember faces, we re-engage the same perceptual processes as we use to identify people. Due to his poor encoding of facial configurations, John is impaired at re-engaging appropriate mechanisms when he tries to recall what people look like – there is a common problem with perception and memory. We will return to this idea in Chapter 11, when we discuss the long-term consequences of agnosia.

Are faces special?

Although some prosopagnosic patients, like FB with whom we began this chapter, can have a quite selective problem with faces, this was not the case for John. We might think then that his problems can tell us little about the relations between face and object processing, since both his were impaired. Nevertheless, there were aspects of John's performance that were considerably worse with faces than with other stimuli, suggesting at least that faces may impose extra processing demands. An example comes from our study of John's ability to detect 'Thatcherised' stimuli (Figure 8.3) [73]. With faces, we found that John was much worse when the whole stimulus was presented (Figure 8.3 top) relative to when we just gave him the parts that had to be discriminated (Figure 8.3 bottom). We also conducted the formally equivalent task with non-face stimuli – houses (Figure 8.5). John had to decide whether the 'parts' of a house (two windows and a door – similar to the eyes and mouth in a face) were the right way up or inverted. These parts were either presented in 'whole house' stimuli (Figure 8.5) or in isolation. With these stimuli, John was no longer impaired for the 'whole' relative to the 'part' displays – this result occurred only with faces. The disruptive effects of the holistic stimulus were more apparent with faces than with other objects [73].

One further test of whether faces were especially difficult for John involved comparing his ability to associate names with faces and with the highly similar class of objects known as 'Greebles', which we introduced in Chapter 4 (see Figure 4.19). We assembled a set of 10 Greebles which differed in terms of how their features were arranged, plus a set of 10 unfamiliar faces (all male). In one block of trials we presented each face for a second and pronounced a name. After giving each of the 10 faces a

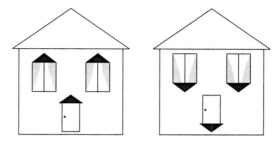

Figure 8.5 Example stimuli from a task requiring judgements as to whether the internal parts of the house (the windows and door) were their correct orientation or inverted. These parts were presented either in isolation or within the 'whole' house.

Source: Reprinted from Boutsen, L. and Humphreys, G. W. Face context interferes with local part processing in a prosopagnosic patient. *Neuropsychologia* 40: 2305–2313 (2002), with permission from Elsevier.

name, we then randomly ordered the stimuli and presented the faces by themselves. John was asked to remember each name. If he was unable to remember all of the names for the faces, we then repeated the initial procedure (giving each face along with its name), and we tested his ability to remember the names again. This procedure was repeated until all of the faces were named correctly. The same protocol was carried out with the Greebles – assigning each a name and then showing each Greeble and requiring John to remember the name. A group of 10 control participants, age-matched to John, were all able to identify all the faces after six learning trials. It was more difficult to learn the names for the Greebles, but they all achieved this after nine learning trials. John was worse than the controls at learning names for each class of stimulus. However, he was able to achieve naming for the Greebles after 18 learning trials. In contrast, he found it impossible to learn the names for the faces and we abandoned the test after 30 trials.

Thus, though control participants found it easier to assign names to faces than to Greebles, John was better at assigning names to Greebles. This result indicates that John found it especially difficult to process and, in this case, form memories for faces compared with other complex stimuli composed of similar parts. The evidence fits with the idea that there are specialised brain regions for processing faces that are damaged in John, and this leads to him having difficulties in face recognition over and above the problems he also has with objects.

Implicit recognition?

Although, by definition, prosopagnosics are impaired at identifying faces, there is remarkable evidence that some patients do access their stored knowledge about faces, but still cannot use this to 'explicitly' know who the individual person. This has been termed 'implicit' recognition [79]. Implicit recognition is judged to occur when knowledge about a person influences another task, even when the person cannot be explicitly named or even (sometimes) discriminated as familiar or not. An example of this comes from studies of face–name learning. Studies have been conducted in which prosopagnosic patients are required to associate names to familiar faces, and the names can either be correct or incorrect (see Figure 8.6). Implicit recognition is shown when the patients are faster to learn the correct pairings (Margaret Thatcher labelled as Margaret Thatcher) compared with the incorrect associations (Margaret Thatcher labelled as Marilyn Monroe) [79]. This pattern of performance is consistent with the faces 'implicitly' activating stored knowledge about the people (otherwise correct and incorrect face–name associations should be learned equally quickly).

We tested for implicit face recognition in John using this same face–name learning procedure. We presented John with sets of three correct face–name pairings and three incorrect pairings. He was given each face and name, and then had to recall the name when shown the face. This procedure was repeated until John could name all the faces across three consecutive trials. He took 14 trials to learn the face–name associations and there was no difference between the correct and incorrect face–name pairings. Although we repeated this test on three different occasions, with different familiar faces, we were never able to show that the correct face–name pairings were learned any better than the incorrect

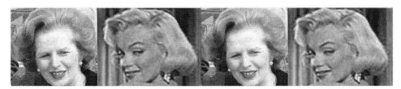

Margaret Thatcher   Marilyn Monroe   Marilyn Monroe   Margaret Thatcher

Figure 8.6 Example stimuli where the face is either paired with the correct name (left and centre left stimuli) or an incorrect name (centre right and right stimuli). Even when patients are unable to explicitly identify the faces, there can be better new learning of correct than incorrect face–name associations.

pairings. We conclude that John's perceptual problems in processing in faces prevented stored knowledge from being strongly activated, and hence recognition could not be demonstrated even using 'implicit' methods. We note that a similar conclusion to this can be drawn from our studies of object processing. In Chapter 7, we discussed studies of shape matching where we presented distractors that belonged to the same category as targets (Figure 7.5) [69]. Normal subjects are slow to reject these distractors compared with distractors coming from a different category to targets – a result indicating implicit recognition of the distractors. John did not show this effect, just as he did not show an advantage for learning correct over incorrect face–name pairings. With faces and objects alike, John's deficit disrupted access to stored knowledge.

Conclusion

John was severely prosopagnosic and his problems with faces surpassed even his problem with objects since he was unable to identify *any* familiar people by sight and he was worse at equivalent tasks with faces compared with objects [73]. Notably John was poor at responding to configural information based on the relations between the internal features of faces, and, indeed, the configural information even seemed to disrupt his performance. This affected John's ability to identify faces and to judge facial emotion and there was no evidence for him accessing stored knowledge about faces implicitly. However, John was able to judge emotion from facial motion and he was better at matching moving than static faces, even when the patterns of movement varied across the matching faces. The results are consistent with faces being processed using different brain mechanisms, depending on, for example, whether the faces are static or moving. John was very impaired at deriving configural information from static facial features and this affected his judgements of facial emotion as well as facial identity. However, he still seemed able to compute the 'biological motion' from faces, when the faces moved, and this enabled him to by-pass the problems in processing static configurations. There was no evidence for implicit recognition.

Notes

1 Eric Morecambe was a UK comedian.
2 Joan Collins and Barbara Windsor are both British actresses. Control participants consistently cite Joan Collins as looking more like Elizabeth Taylor, given this choice.

Chapter 9

Colour, movement, action!

I can't tell you its colour but it has a strong reflectance.

(John)

Seeing colour

John's job had involved him working in art galleries and museums advising on coverings to minimise deterioration in the condition of precious objets d'art. He knew a lot about colours – which were likely to be bright, which dark, under different lighting conditions – and he depended on colour vision for his livelihood. However, after his stroke, he lost all subjective impression of colour and described the world as being in shades of grey. John's lesion compromised area V4 in the ventral visual stream of the brain – a region thought to be crucial for colour perception [4, 8]. It was not surprising then that he was 'achromatopsic' – that is, cortically colour blind. Similar to his problems in object recognition, this was not simply an impairment in finding the name for colours – he had problems in matching colours too. We showed him sets of colour patches from a series of paints – one set of patches was placed in front of him and another, with the patches in a different order, in front of us. We pointed to one patch and he had to point to the matching colour in his set. He made many errors – typically pointing to a colour close to the one we were pointing to. He never made an error by pointing to a dark colour when we pointed to a light one, but the ability to make fine distinctions within a colour range appeared to be poor.

We examined this more formally using a test called the Farnsworth-Munsell 100 hue test, where the task is to arrange colours swatches in either an ascending or descending order of colour. Importantly, the colours in each set are matched for brightness, so the ordering must be based on colour discrimination not the relative lightness or darkness of the stimuli.

Again John was impaired at ordering the colour swatches, making errors that would not be found in someone with good colour perception [80].

Was there any evidence of some preservation of his colour processing? We evaluated this by giving John two 'random noise' patches and he just had to judge whether the patches were the same or whether they differed (see Figure 9.1 in the plate section) [81]. Within each patch, the 'pixels' could have the same or different brightnesses and colours, which created three conditions: the patches could differ in colour but be the same brightness, they could have the same colour but differ in brightness or they could differ in both colour and brightness. The task was to judge whether the two patches were the same or different.

John was above chance at making these judgements, even when the stimuli only differed in colour. Thus there was some evidence of some preservation of colour processing, though John was subjectively unaware of it. We then added 'dynamic luminance noise' to the displays, by having pixels flicker at different rates. The idea was that the normal colour perception system, based on parvocellular neurons, has a slow response and is relatively insensitive to rapid dynamic change. In contrast, the dynamic magnocellular system – which may still carry some differential response to contrasting colours – would be 'swamped' by the dynamic luminance noise. If the dynamic system was being used by John, then performance should drop dramatically when dynamic noise is present. We found that John was quite impervious to this dynamic noise, although another achromatopsic patient tested along with John was strongly affected – for this last patient any residual ability to tell the difference between the contrasting colour patches had been lost [81]. The two patterns of results indicate that, in John, the slow-acting colour-sensitive neurons, normally dominant for our colour perception, continued to act – albeit that they did not convey enough information for John to be able to explicitly see colour. The second achromatopsic patient, however, seemed to be using the residual capacities of a motion-based processing system – and so was strongly disrupted by dynamic noise.

Given that John was impaired at colour perception, was his memory for colour also affected? Our study of John's ability to remember faces indicated some commonality between his perception and his memory for faces – perhaps the same also held for colour? In pursuit of this question, we asked John to name the colours associated with different objects which have consistent colour associations [58], for example:

What colour is a radish?
What colour is a watermelon?

We also included questions where the colour was less visually and more conceptually related to the item, for example:

> What colour is associated with jealousy?
> What colour of gold is used to describe oil?

John performed well with the more abstract questions about colour – there was no problem in producing the name 'green' associated with jealousy. However, he was less good at naming colours that required more visual knowledge – perhaps re-picturing the object [58]. The result again points to an association between perception and memory, with John's perceptual problem with colour also affecting – specifically – his visual memory for colour. Conceptual knowledge about colour was relatively spared (e.g., John knew that oil was known as black gold, etc.).

We examined whether the residual colour information that John had could influence how well he recognised objects. We presented John with black-and-white line drawings of objects, correctly coloured drawings and drawings that were given the incorrect colours for the objects. If colour helped his recognition, we would expect his identification to be best when the objects were coloured correctly. What we found differed from this. He was better at identifying correctly coloured line drawings than black-and-white drawings. However, the correctly coloured drawings were no better than the incorrectly coloured drawings, and these too were identified more accurately than black-and-white drawings. The result was clear. John was helped by colouring the surfaces of objects, which reduced his tendency to make segmentation errors, grouping together the wrong parts of objects. In contrast, there was no influence of whether the object carried the correct or the incorrect colour – colour did not directly affect his access to stored knowledge [82].

Seeing depth

In contrast to his poor colour perception, John retained a good ability to perceive other basic aspects of visual stimuli – such as their depth. To some degree, this was apparent from observing John's actions in everyday life, where he would reach to objects efficiently and negotiate obstacles without any apparent problems. Depth information can be conveyed through a variety of cues. Binocular depth cues are provided by the differences in the positions of stimuli in each eye (try closing one eye and then the other to notice the shift in the position of the image for objects close to you). The brain is able to use these differences in image position (the 'binocular disparity') to compute the relative distances of objects – at least for objects falling around an arm's length away from us (for objects further away than this, the position shifts become too slight to provide useful information about depth). Bela Julesz [83] designed special stimuli to demonstrate that binocular disparity on its own can be used to 'see' depth. These 'random dot stereograms' were composed of patches of pixels with random brightness – similar to the patches presented in Figure 9.1. The two patches were identical apart from one section, which was shifted in one direction in one patch relative to the other. When each patch is seen alone, the shifted section cannot be seen because it is just another area of random pattern. However, if one patch is presented to one eye and the second patch to the other, then the brain is able to compare the stimuli coming to each eye and to compute that the images match apart from the shifted section. This shifted section is then interpreted as differing in depth from the non-shifted section – it is seen either floating above or below the non-shifted section (depending on the direction of the shift). Here the brain has only the binocular disparity between the images to work with, but it is nevertheless able to use this to create the impression of two surfaces, one in front of the other (the shifted section and the remaining areas which match in the images). This ability is termed stereopsis. We gave random dot stereograms of this type to John and he had no difficulty in being able to discriminate the shape that had been shifted, whether it protruded from or fell behind the surrounding context and where it appeared in the field. John had good stereopsis.

As well as being able to judge depth from binocular disparities, there are multiple other cues to depth present when we move around the world. For example, there are linear perspective cues as edges recede to the point at which we fixate, there are relative size cues (as objects that are more distant occupy less of the image), and there are 'motion parallax' cues (when we move our heads, objects that are close move at a different rate to objects that are further away). All of these depth cues are used when we negotiate our environment and interact with objects. They may also be used when we recognise objects, especially if other visual information is degraded.

We tested if John used these different depth cues to aid his object recognition [82]. Similar to previously reported patients with agnosia, John was better at identifying real objects than line drawings – he was typically able to identify about 60 per cent of common household objects shown one at a time under good lighting conditions, but he was only able to name about 40 per cent of the same items when they were depicted as line drawings. We had John view real objects and line drawings either seen within reaching distance (when strong binocular depth cues are present) or at a farther distance (with weakened binocular depth cues). In addition, he was allowed to make free head movements or we restricted his head movements by having him place his chin in a 'chin rest'. The advantage for real objects over line drawings was greatest when either binocular depth cues were present (objects within reaching distance) or when he could use motion parallax (with free head movements), but the advantage receded when the depth cues were reduced (with objects shown at a distance and head movements restricted).

The presence of depth cues helped John 'parse' the object into its correct parts and surfaces. This was demonstrated by having him copy the stimuli in these different depth conditions. Figure 9.2 shows examples of the real objects and line drawings that John was presented along with

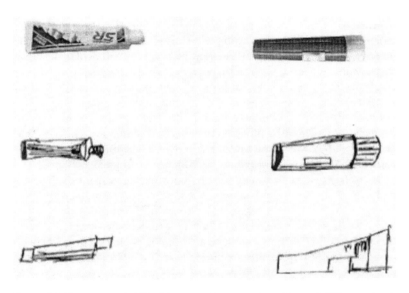

Figure 9.2 Top: example 3D objects used to test the effects of different depth cues on John's object recognition. Middle: John's drawings of these objects in the 'distant free' condition (objects presented at a distance but free head movements allowed). Bottom: John's drawings of the same objects in the 'distant, fixed' condition (objects presented at a distance but with his head fixed).

Source: From Chainay, H. and Humphreys, G. W. (2001). The real-object advantage in agnosia: evidence for a role of surface and depth information in object recognition. *Cognitive Neuropsychology* 18: 175–191, reprinted by permission of the publisher (Taylor & Francis Group, http://www.informaworld.com).

his copies of the stimuli in the different viewing conditions. When the depth cues were restricted (in the 'fixed, distant' condition), John's drawings betrayed his incorrect 'parsing' of the part of complex objects – in this case, parts were not always correctly grouped together. The depth cues provided additional information to guide his encoding and grouping of object parts by informing him about which parts fell in front of others. The results indicate that an important factor in John's improved recognition of real objects over line drawings was the presence of depth cues when he encountered real objects.

Reaching, grasping and 'affordance'

As well as being able to employ depth information to better recognise objects, John also showed good use of depth information in how he acted in his environment. There were no pronounced problems in negotiating stairs beyond becoming increasing stiff in his movements as he grew older. He could walk around objects and he could reach and grasp objects with a fluency that matched that in other subjects of the same age – the velocity and trajectory of the motion, the opening of his hand prior to it reaching the objects, all the components of the action were spared. We also assessed him on a test where patients with poor visuo-motor co-ordination have great difficulty – which involves having the patient 'post' a flat visual card through a 'letter box' which can be angled at different orientations (see Figure 9.3). Patients with poor visuo-motor co-ordination find it difficult to align the card with the angle of the letter box [84]. John had no difficulty doing this though, and he moved without hesitation to post the card each time we tested him.

However, John did betray one problem in using vision for action – which was that he might reach and grasp the wrong part of an object (e.g., reaching to the blade of a knife because he mistook it for the handle!). This aspect of action may depend on access to stored knowledge about the object, not just on access to visual information about which part is potentially graspable based on its 'low-level' properties (e.g., its coarse global shape). In this case, John's ability to act upon objects was limited. The contrast between visual misidentification and a good ability to carry out basic reaching and grasping actions has motivated the argument that 'vision for action' is distinct from 'vision for recognition' – with 'vision for action' taking place along the dorsal visual route and 'vision for recognition' being supported by the ventral visual route [84]. John had a spared dorsal visual route and a damaged ventral route, and his behaviour is consistent with this 'action vs. recognition' distinction.

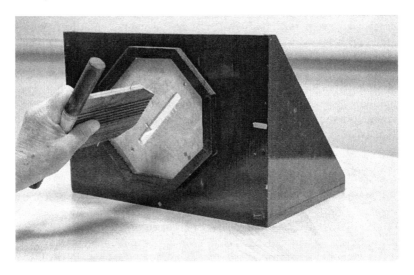

Figure 9.3 Example stimuli from the 'letter posting' task. John was asked to take the card (shown here in the actor's hand) and to post it through the slot in the apparatus in front of him. We measured the speed and accuracy with which he did this. There was no difference between John's performance and that of control participants.

We also tested whether John's ability to recognise objects was affected by whether the objects might be strongly associated with action. To do this we used an experimental procedure introduced by Tucker and Ellis [85]. Tucker and Ellis had normal subjects make a right or left button press response according to whether an implement was shown upright or upside down (Figure 9.4). In addition, the implement could have its handle turned to the right or left. When the handle was turned to the right, then responses made with the right hand were speeded (sometimes this might be to respond that the object was upright, sometimes that it was inverted – depending on which decision was linked to the right hand response). When the handle was turned to the left, then responses with the left hand were speeded. To explain these data, Tucker and Ellis invoked an idea put forward by the ecological psychologist James Gibson [86]. Gibson proposed that our perceptual systems are tuned to 'affordances' – action-related properties of our environment. Essentially, an implement with its handle turned to the right generates an affordance to make a right hand response, and this leads to faster responses with the right hand (and similarly faster responses with the left hand when the handle is turned to the left). We tested John with a set of implements, some of which he could and some of which he could not identify. Interestingly, when we presented the same items to normal participants and asked them to respond according to whether the objects were upright or inverted, we found that the objects that produced the largest 'affordance effect' (i.e., speeded responses when the hand of response matched the side of the handle) were also the objects that John could identify. Using just these objects we also observed that, like the control participants, John produced an 'affordance effect' – but in his case the effect was around four times bigger than that produced by the controls, even when we took any differences in overall response speed into account. These intriguing data suggest two things. One is that John was more strongly affected by affordance than normal participants. The second is that his ability to identify objects was itself at least partly influenced by the affordance conveyed by the object. Both results fit with the proposal of two visual routes in the brain, and with John's dorsal (action) route being spared while his ventral (recognition) route is lesioned. Due to the damage to the ventral route, responses triggered through the dorsal route are dominant and may even support his object identification.

We might then ask about what properties of objects are used by the dorsal action route. Here we note that the affordance we manipulated was very simple (whether a handle was facing left or right) and was likely to be conveyed by the general outline of the object – which we know that

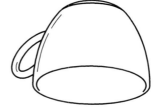

Figure 9.4 Example stimuli from the study of 'affordance effect' with John. A right-hand response might have to be made to an upright object (left) and a left-hand response to an inverted object (right). Right hand responses were speeded when the handle faced to the right and left hand responses were speeded when the handle faced to the left.

Source: From Snodgrass, J. G. and Vanderwart, M. A. (1980) A standardised set of 260 pictures: norms for name agreement, familiarity and name complexity. *Journal of Experimental Psychology: Human Learning and Memory* 6: 174–215.

John could respond to (see Chapter 7). Rather than thinking that the dorsal action route was using information not available to John's (ventral) recognition system, we think it more likely that both routes had access to the same incoming information, but this could be used by the dorsal route to trigger action-related responses. Indeed, as we have noted, John was liable to pick up objects by the wrong part when he failed to recognise them – a knife by the blade, for example. This indicates that the dorsal route did not provide any more information than the ventral route about which was the correct part of the object to grasp.

Seeing motion

Our early tests with John indicated that his ability to perceive motion, like the perception of depth, remained intact. John had no problems in following a pen with his eyes, when his ability to make 'smooth pursuit' eye movement was tested [58]. If thrown a tennis ball, he could catch it. If a ball was rolled along a table, he was able to stop it at the appropriate time before it fell. John's motion perception was evaluated more formally by presenting him with two moving stimuli and having him decide which moved faster or whether they moved in the same direction. His performance was the equal of that of control participants of a similar age.

We also tested whether John could use motion cues to help him 'parse' visual displays – the root cause of his problem in recognising static objects (see Chapter 7). We had John search for a target letter (e.g., is an N present?) presented among other randomly selected letters – a task that normally involves scanning each letter until the target is found. In one case all the letters were presented together and either remained in the same place (the static condition) or they all moved together across the display. In the critical condition, half the distractor letters were static and half moved. On different trial blocks the target (the N) was always stationary or it always moved. An example display is depicted in Figure 9.5.

Control participants find it much easier to find the target when half the distractors move and half are static, compared with when they are all stationary or all move together. Here the presence of common motion for one set of items enables these items to be segmented from the others – it is almost as if the moving and static items occupy two different 'plains' in depth, with it then being possible to attend to one plain while ignoring the other. We found the same results for John. John had a perfect ability to 'filter out' the irrelevant items – shown by his search rate being halved when half of distractors moved compared to when all the distractors

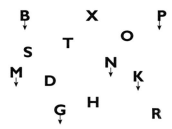

Figure 9.5 An example of the visual search task. The target was always the letter N which could be stationary or moving (in this example, the N is moving downwards) presented among other randomly selected letters. In the critical condition, half the distractor letters were static and half moved (as indicated by the presence or absence of arrows).

moved or were static. The results indicate that John only searched the moving or static group containing the target, and the irrelevant group had no impact on his performance.

These results indicate that John could use motion to help segment relevant from irrelevant parts of an image. This contrasts with his very impaired ability to segment displays based on static forms (see Chapter 7). We conclude that distinct brain processes mediate segmentation using static form information and segmentation using motion, and that the latter processes were spared in John's case. This is consistent with motion processing being supported by more dorsal regions of the cortical visual system (e.g., area MT, Figure 4.1), which were not affected by his lesion.

Navigation

It is one thing to see objects in depth and as they move, and to be able to reach and grasp those within reach; it is another thing to use this visual information to navigate your environment. As both John and Iris remarked on at the initial time after his stroke, John was remarkably poor at finding his way. Despite tracing out a route many times, John was still very prone to become lost, especially if distracted along the way. Initially we construed the problem in route finding as a reflection of the same fundamental deficit as that underlying John's agnosia for objects – after all it must be extremely difficult to recognise where you are if you cannot recognise particular landmarks [87]. However, further analysis indicated that the problem was not simply one of poor object recognition.

John could get lost within his home, despite experiencing this limited environment every day and despite being able to recognise the familiar objects present. To try and understand this difficulty in navigating the environment we asked John to copy and then draw his room from memory [88]. At this time John had moved to sheltered accommodation and spent a good deal of his time in this one room. We were sure he could identify all of the major items in the room, as he both felt and saw them every day. Figure 9.6 presents his drawings. Figure 9.6(b) represents John's copying of the layout of the furniture in the room. Figure 9.6(a) is his drawing from memory taken about 10 minutes after he had left the room. What can be seen from his drawing from memory is that, not only were items omitted, but also that he mislocated items, for example,

(a)

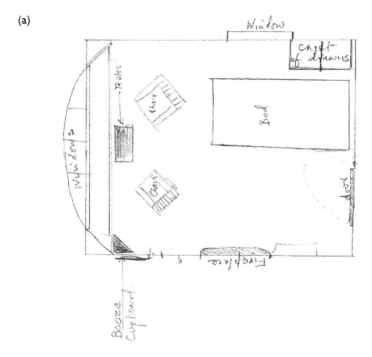

Figure 9.6 John's drawings of his room: (a) drawn after leaving the room for 10 min.; (b) direct copy of the room; (c) one year after leaving the home

Source: From Riddoch, M. J. et al. (2003). Visual and spatial short-term memory in visual agnosia. *Cognitive Neuropsychology* 20: 641–671, reprinted by permission of the publisher (Taylor & Francis Group, http://www.informaworld. com).

(b)

PLEASE STAND IN THE DOORWAY OF YOUR BEDROOM, LOOKING INTO THE ROOM.

DRAW (AND LABEL) THE POSITIONS OF ALL ITEMS OF FURNITURE (INCLUDING WINDOWS AND DOORS).

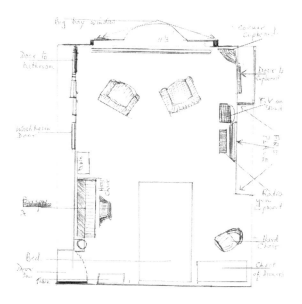

(c)

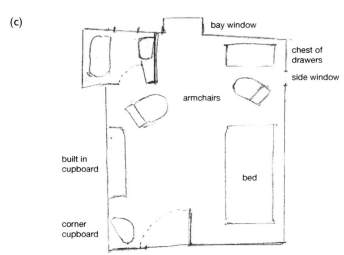

Figure 9.6 continued

putting the fireplace on the wrong side of the room in relation to the window. Figure 9.6(c) gives his drawing from long-term memory. This drawing was executed about one year after John had left the first residential home and moved to another. Again he reproduced only a limited number of objects and he again shifted the relative positions of the objects within the room – the bed was positioned fully into the corner, a chest of drawers was repositioned in relation to the window, etc. This was not because the furniture had been re-positioned, as the furniture remained in the same locations throughout John's tenure. It was really that John had a poor internal representation of the relative locations of objects even within this very familiar environment.

This difficulty was not confined to familiar environments but extended to tasks requiring him to judge the relative locations of cities in the UK. For example, John reported that to go from London to Bristol involved going due north, when it is due west. Given that John travelled frequently across the UK as part of his job, had been a pilot etc., it is unlikely that he had not had this geographic knowledge at one stage. We suggest instead that John was poor at representing the co-locations of a number of separate objects on a large-scale 'mental map'. This was not simply a problem in visual memory or in manipulating a mental image. We gave him an imagery task requiring the mental manipulation of letters. For example, imagine a capital D. Now turn it through 90 degrees to the left. Now take a capital J and move it underneath the D. What object does this make? (Answer: an umbrella.) With this task John performed at the same level as you or I. We conclude that there was not a general problem in imagery but a more specific one in representing the relations between objects over a larger scale. In Chapter 4 we discussed data from functional imaging drawing a distinction between brain activity in the LOC which is sensitive to the relations between objects, and the parahippocampal gyrus, which is responsive to overall scene structure but not the identities of individual objects [24]. John's lesions extended to the parahippocampal gyri in both hemispheres and consequently could have affected his ability to use overall scene structure to help relate objects to one another. This problem in co-locating objects could occur over and above the perceptual impairments that led to poor recognition of single objects – and, indeed, it occurred with tasks such as drawing his room arrangements from memory, which are not contingent on individual object recognition.

Conclusion

The studies show that John's ability to process visual features varied. His perception of colour was impaired. However, he had a good ability to see in depth, and information about the relative depths of surfaces helped him 'parse' objects correctly, supporting visual object identification. In addition, and as long as the task did not depend on object identification, John was able to reach and grasp objects appropriately; he also responded to action-related properties of objects ('affordances'). He could use motion information when interacting with the world and motion could be employed to segment relevant from irrelevant parts of an image. These results fit with the framework we are proposing, that there is decomposition of different visual features by the brain within contrasting cortical regions, and that some features (such as depth and motion) can be used to compensate for impairments in integrating visual form. In addition, John had marked problems in recognising his environment, and this problem occurred even under conditions in which he recognised the individual objects present. To explain this last result, we suggest that John suffered a separate and specific deficit in representing objects in a large-scale scene structure, a process normally subserved by the parahippocampal gyri, which were lesioned in his case.

Chapter 10

The written word

If I can immediately remember what I've written, it helps, otherwise I am lost.

(John)

Alexia

Once you have learned to read fluently as a child, reading usually proceeds very efficiently – so efficiently in fact that it can be difficult to prevent. Perhaps the best known example of this is the 'Stroop' effect, named after John Ridley Stroop who first reported data on this in a paper in 1935 [89]. Stroop gave participants colour words presented in different colours (e.g., the word BLUE printed in the colour red or blue) and asked them to name either the colours or the words. Word naming was little affected by whether the colours were matched to the words, whereas colour naming was strongly affected by whether the words matched the colours: colour naming was much easier if the words matched the colours (the colour blue applied to the word BLUE or the colour red applied to the word RED) than if the words were incongruent with the colours (the colour red applied to the word BLUE or the colour blue to the word RED). The selective interference from the word on colour naming is usually attributed to the word being read rapidly and automatically, with the word name then competing with the colour name for the response that participants must make.

As well as word reading being apparently automatic, it also seems to be based on visual processes that take in multiple letters together, so that the time to name words is little affected by the number of letters present – at least for words with up to six or seven letters. This efficient reading of words contrasts with the ability of patients to read after damage to the ventral visual stream in posterior regions of the left hemisphere. After damage to the left ventral regions, patients can experience severe difficulties in reading – sometimes only being able to read words by first generating the sounds associated with each letter. This disorder was first documented by a French neurologist, Dejerine, in 1892 [90] and it was termed 'alexia' – referring to an inability to read whole words. As was the case with John, the disorder can arise even when patients may be able to spell words from memory – when it is then labelled as 'alexia without agraphia'.

Alexia is typically diagnosed by presenting patients with words of different lengths and requiring them to name the words as quickly as they can. Normally, reaction times to name the words increase little as the number of letters in the words increases – and even when words with more than six letters are presented, the time to read the words increases by less than one-tenth of a second (100 ms) for each extra letter present. We evaluated this in John by giving him words made up of three, five or seven letters. Although the words tested at each length were equally frequent and all referred to concrete concepts, his time to name the words went from ~1.5 sec. to over 3.75 sec. as the letter length increased – that is, there was an extra cost of over half a second (500 ms) for every extra letter that was added (Figure 10.1). This was over five times the effect of word length found in control participants of a similar age to John. Also, when compared with the age-matched controls, John was much more variable in his reading – sometimes taking a relatively long time to read short words or a relatively short time to read longer words (indicated by the size of the errors bars on the graphs shown in Figure 10.1 – the

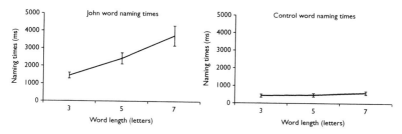

Figure 10.1 Mean times to name words by John (left) and age-matched control participants (right). The bars show the standard deviation in naming times across the words at each length. Note that John was overall much slower, he was more affected by the length of the words and he was more variable across the words. Note that 1000ms =1 sec. It took John around 2 sec. to read a 3-letter word and around 4 sec., twice as long, to read a word with 7 letters.

bigger the error bar, the greater the variability). This variability in reading times has been noted previously in alexic patients [91].

The abnormally strong effects of word length found in alexic patients has led to them being labelled as 'letter-by-letter readers', suggesting that the patients are only able to read words after serially identifying each letter – hence the longer the words, the more time is required to name them. One account of the disorder is that alexic patients have lost the 'visual word form system', normally present in the left ventral cortex (see Chapter 4, Figure 4.20), and so they can no longer recognise words as a single 'visual unit'. Lacking a visual word form system, the patients must fall back on identifying each letter in turn to eventually read a word [36].

However, there are reasons to question whether this is the whole story. For example, consider the task of reading words whose letters are presented in MiXeD cAsE. If a patient is simply reading each letter in turn, and if there is little difference in the time taken to name upper case and lower case letters, then they should be able to read MiXeD cAsE words as efficiently as words written in just one case (single CASE). Surprisingly, this is not what happens – such patients frequently find MiXeD cAsE words much harder to read than words written in just one case, and this effect is also much larger than is found with normal readers [92]. MiXeD case words, of course, look less familiar overall than words written in a single case. The vulnerability of alexic patients to CaSe MiXiNg suggests that they may be sensitive to the overall look of words, and not simply reading them letter-by-letter. Our results with John fit this argument. As shown in Figure 10.2, John was greatly slowed when he had to read MiXeD cAsE words compared with words written in either UPPER or lower case; the controls showed a much smaller effect.

In another test of whether John was really reading letter-by-letter, we contrasted his performance when all the letters of the words were presented together and when we presented one letter at a time, but at a rate we calculated from how much his naming times increased as each additional letter was added to words (this can be estimated from the slope of the graph for John presented in Figure 10.1; in this case, we presented each letter for 0.5 sec. at a time). We then compared how quickly John could name words when all the letters were presented together (the complete word condition) and when the letters appeared sequentially [93]. Here we might expect that his naming times might be equal in these two conditions, if he was identifying the words by sequentially identifying the letters. In contrast to this prediction, John was much faster to read words when the letters were presented sequentially compared to

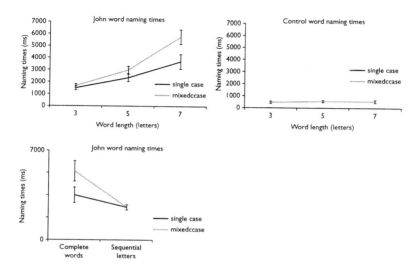

Figure 10.2 Mean naming times by John (a) and age-matched control participants (b) to words written in single case (UPPER or lower) or in MiXeD cAsE. Note the much greater slowing of naming for John than for the controls when the words appeared in MiXeD cAsE. (c) Mean naming times for John to read complete words and words presented as a series of letters in single and MiXeD case. Note that there was no effect of CaSe MiXiNg when letters were presented sequentially.

when they all appeared together – his naming times reduced by one-third in the sequential condition. Exactly the opposite results occurred for the control participants. The controls were faster to name words when all the letters appeared together compared to when the letters were presented sequentially (again using presentation rates matched to the estimated speed of reading the letters, in the complete word condition).

These opposite effects of complete and sequential presentation of words can be understood if, normally, we benefit from having all the letters in words presented together, precisely because the words are processed and recognised as a single visual unit; breaking up the unit (presenting one letter at a time) eliminates the gains from processing all the letters together. In direct contrast to this, John's better reading in the sequential condition suggests that he finds the complete words disruptive – slowing his reading compared to when each letter appears alone. That is, John does not simply read letter-by-letter – rather he processes the multiple letters in the word but his processing of the multiple letters breaks down, leading to reading that is slower than you would expect from 'pure' serial letter identification.

A further striking result occurred when we combined the manipulations of CaSe MiXiNg and whether we presented complete words or each word as a sequence of letters. When complete words were presented, there were again strong effects of CaSe MiXiNg – naming times were much slower when the letters alternated in case – however, this effect vanished when the letters were presented sequentially. Thus, when John was forced to read letter-by-letter, when the letters were presented sequentially, the effects of CaSe MiXiNg disappeared. This indicates that the effects of CaSe MiXiNg were confined to when John attempted to process all the letters together. The results suggest that John was affected by the visual complexity of complete words, and was much more disrupted than normal when the visual familiarity decreased through CaSe MiXiNg. One account of this is that CaSe MiXiNg adds 'noise' to the representation of the complete word, and John was abnormally affected by this extra visual noise.

Consider now the variability in John's reading time across different words (Figures 10.1 and 10.2), which was much larger than that found in normal readers. This variability would arise if John's processing of complete words was visually 'noisy', with the noise level varying across different occasions – with the result that there is variability in naming times. The variability also suggests that John has not simply lost his 'visual word form system'; rather the system is operating but in a noisy manner. These results on John's reading, where he is sensitive to visual information in complete words, are reminiscent of his object and face recognition. Concerning John's object and face recognition we have argued that he processes complete shapes and facial configurations, but the representations coded are coarse and noisy and fail to serve the more precise recognition of individual objects (see Chapter 6). We can make a similar argument concerning his reading. We suggest that John had noisy global representations of words, but these representations were not complemented by more detailed information about the local parts (here the letters in words). Lacking this more detailed information at a global level, he fell back on sequential, parts-based recognition (here letter-by-letter reading).

Agnosia, alexia, prosopagnosia

As we have discussed in Chapters 6–8 and also in this chapter, John's brain lesions disrupted his object recognition, his reading and his face recognition, rendering him agnosic, alexic and prosopagnosic. Martha Farah, from the University of Pennsylvania, reviewed evidence on the relations between these three disorders in her book, *Visual Agnosia* [94, 95]. She argued that, historically, cases had been reported with 'pure alexia' (a problem in reading without difficulties in object and face recognition) and 'pure prosopagnosia' (a problem in face recognition without difficulties in object recognition and reading), but not 'pure agnosia' without there being some concomitant problem in either reading or face recognition. From this selective grouping of the deficits she suggested that there were fundamentally two types of visual coding: a holistic 'non-decomposed' coding of objects and a parts-based coding of the multiple elements making up stimuli. She argued that faces were supported by holistic coding and word recognition was supported by parts-based coding, whereas object recognition could vary according to whether holistic or parts-based coding was more strongly weighted for the particular stimulus. A selective brain lesion that disrupted holistic coding alone could lead to 'pure prosopagnosia' without major impact on objects or words. A lesion that impaired parts-based coding alone would affect reading but not face recognition. If either lesion was more extensive, then object recognition too might be affected, and this might vary according to whether the object depended on holistic or parts-based recognition. A framework illustrating these ideas is presented in Figure 10.3.

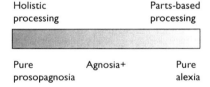

Figure 10.3 An analysis of the relations between agnosia, alexia and prosopagnosia presented by Martha Farah (1990 and 2004). According to this framework, a deficit in holistic processing should result in pure prosopagnosia, while a deficit in parts-based processing will result in pure alexia. When the holistic and parts-based deficits are more widespread, object recognition will be impaired (resulting in agnosia). A widespread impairment in holistic processing will produce agnosia + prosopagnosia; a widespread deficit in parts-based processing will generate agnosia + alexia.

Source: Farah, M. J. (1990) *Visual Agnosia*. Cambridge, MA: MIT Press; Farah, M. J. (2004) *Visual Agnosia*, 2nd edn. Cambridge, MA: MIT Press, reprinted by permission of the publisher (Taylor & Francis Group, http://www.informa world.com).

This is an elegant account of the relations between the visual processes serving face, object and word recognition, linking neuropsychological disorders of each task back to impairments in two fundamental processes. Unfortunately, things are not quite as straight-forward. For example, this account predicts that it should not be possible for a patient to be prosopagnosic and alexic without also having visual agnosia – since this would mean that they had impaired holistic and parts-based processes, and object recognition should suffer accordingly. In addition, it should not be possible for a patient to have agnosia without also having an associated problems in either face or word recognition, since the agnosia would reflect either a problem in holistic or in parts-based recognition, and this should in turn disrupt face recognition or reading respectively. These predictions turn out to be incorrect. Buxbaum and colleagues [96] reported a patient who read aloud in a letter-by-letter fashion and who failed to identify the faces of famous people yet who was not agnosic and readily identified real objects. That is, alexia and proposagnosia without agnosia was observed. Contrasting with this, we have described two individuals who were agnosic (e.g., being poor not only at naming objects but also at deciding whether pairs of objects were related to one another) but who were good at identifying faces and who could read words well too (including reading English words that have irregular relations between their spelling and their sound – such words are difficult to name without first being recognised as a familiar word). These then were cases of agnosia without alexia and prosopagnosia [97, 98]. The cases that counter the 'two processes' account can be explained if we understand that visual recognition problems can reflect 'memorial' as well as 'perceptual' deficits. For example, both of the cases of 'pure agnosia' (without alexia or prosopagnosia) we reported had problems in stored knowledge about objects. Figure 10.4 gives examples of one patient's drawing from memory of objects (the agnosic patient MH), which was clearly worse than direct copying. We suggest that a 'pure agnosia' can occur when stored knowledge specific to objects is affected. In this case, the problems would not necessarily reflect a perceptual deficit in processing holistic or parts-based visual representations.

However, even this 'memorial' account is not sufficient. Consider John's reading. Here the evidence suggests that he is sensitive to multiple letters in words and he does not adopt a serial parts-based approach of identifying each letter – yet the framework assumes that reading is supported by parts-based recognition. In Chapter 4 we also argued that John was sensitive to holistic representations of objects (e.g., to global shapes rather than the local elements of compound letters) but he had

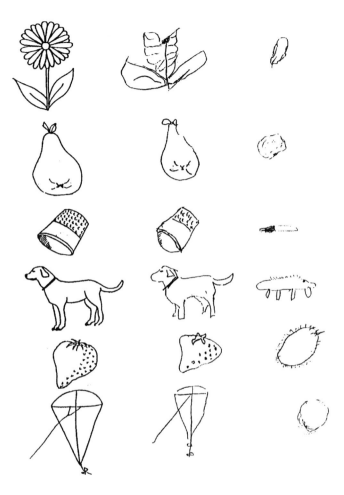

Figure 10.4 Left: exemplar objects that the agnosic patient MH was asked to copy. Centre: examples of MH's copies. Right: examples of MH's drawing from memory of the same objects when he was given each object's name. MH was strikingly poor at remembering the visual characteristics of objects, which was not a problem in drawing – given his accurate copies. MH's poor visual memory contrasts with that of John who initially was very good at remembering what objects looked like (see Chapter 3).

Source: From Humphreys, G. W. and Rumiati, R. I. (1998). Agnosia without prosopagnosia or alexia: evidence for stored visual memories specific to objects. *Cognitive Neuropsychology* 15: 243–277.

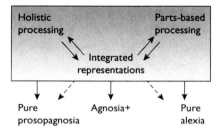

Figure 10.5 A framework for face, object and word recognition in which integrated (holistic representations embellished by information about local parts) contribute to each recognition process

difficulty because these holistic representations were not embellished by local detail. What seems important here is not the coding of holistic and parts-based representations alone, but rather the way in which these representations integrate. We propose that John's impairment lay not in his ability to compute holistic representations or to carry out parts-based analysis – the problem lay in the integration between parts and whole. Accordingly, we present an alternative to the two processes (holistic and parts-based) account we illustrated in Figure 10.3 [94, 95]. This alternative, shown in Figure 10.5, suggests that object recognition is normally dependent on the integration of holistic and parts-based information from stimuli, not the separate coding of wholes and parts. Also the integrated codes feed into both word and face recognition, contributing to these tasks along with the distinct holistic and parts-based processes. On this view, a breakdown in the integration process, which we have suggested was critical to John's agnosia (see Chapters 6 and 7), will affect face, object and word recognition.

Writing

Unlike reading, John found it easy to write. Figure 10.6 present a letter written to us following one test session. Apart from sensing his unfailing politeness and good humour, you can see that John's writing was generally fluent and his spellings were accurate. There were occasional errors. Here he mis-spelled the word 'turn' as 'tern' and he omitted the word 'know' (in turn know how . . .). However such errors were rare and did not occur when he was asked to take one word at a time and spell from memory. We conclude that his 'spelling lexicon' was unaffected by his stroke.

One long-standing question is whether the memories that support visual word recognition are the same as the memories used to support spelling. Cases of alexia without agraphia, such as John, are informative for this debate because they suggest that memory for spellings can be distinct from the memories supporting word recognition – given that such patients can spell but not read. John's case is generally consistent with this view, especially as he was able to write words with irregular spellings which must be produced by memory rather than by translating sounds

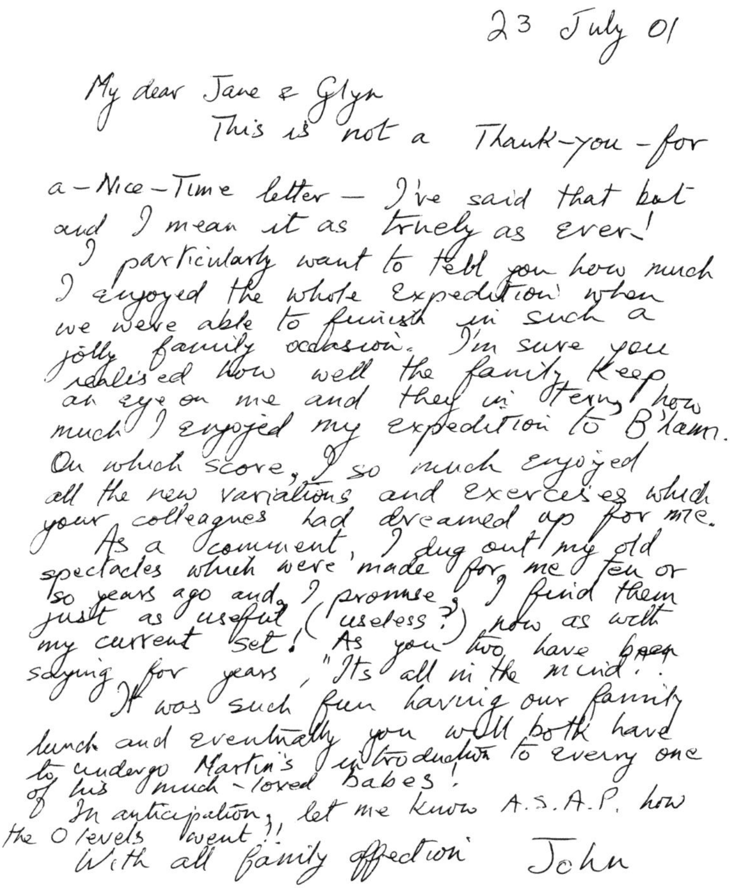

Figure 10.6 An example of John's writing

directly into letters. The one caveat concerns John's visual errors when writing words. These errors suggest that he sometimes consulted his noisy visual recognition system when remembering letter forms, and so generated the wrong letter form. However, this was only done when the form had to be written, whereas his oral spelling was dissociated from his reading.

Conclusion

John showed many of the 'classic' symptoms of alexia without agraphia. He was abnormally affected by word length, being progressively slower to read longer words. He also found MiXeD cAsE words particularly difficult. Strikingly, his word naming was faster when the letters were presented one at a time and the effects of CaSe MiXiNg disappeared under sequential presentation conditions. We conclude that John still processed complete words but that his word representations were noisy and did not support accurate word recognition. In contrast to his reading, his writing was generally good and his oral spelling was accurate even for words that do not follow the spelling-to-sound regularities of English. This last result fits with the idea that reading and spelling rely on different long-term memories for words, and that John has no impairment within his long-term memory for spellings.

Chapter 11

Living with agnosia

Frustration is still my hated driver.

(John)

John lived with agnosia for 26 and a half years before he died in 2008. During this time, he became reconciled to his recognition problems and was much more sanguine about losing his way or misidentifying friends and family than he was in the early days after his stroke. Five years after the stroke, we asked Iris to describe how things had been, from her point of view, taking our questions as prompts. She wrote as follows to our question 'Have there been any changes?'

Yes – possibly the biggest of these is the increase in his self-confidence and acceptance of his limitations. Whereas in the past he would make no effort to tune his radio from one station to another, he will now do it for himself. He can also now manipulate the TV remote control and adjust the level of sound without any help.

He has also gained confidence in the car and is able to relax accepting that the driver can judge speed and distance even if he is unable to.

His reading ability has now improved considerably so now he spends a long time each morning with the newspaper. When he tries to read an extract to me it is at the speed of a child but he manages to invent a few words here and there to get the story told! Unfortunately I have not been able to interest him in reading books – besides the slow reading ability, his poor short-term memory prevents him from remembering what he read the morning or the day before – hence the story, having no continuity, has no interest. However, he can now read labels on some bottles if the print is large and not in 'fancy writing'. This has stopped the confusion between toothpaste and shaving cream and enabled him to select the cassette he wishes to play on his tape recorder. He struggles to read typed letters but hand writing defeats him, although recently I have noticed him slowly reading his own handwriting when he is interrupted in the middle of writing a letter.

Colour remains a tricky problem. I am probably more aware of this than John because he does not see his mistakes or, should I say, my mistakes. If the temperature drops and he goes to select a cardigan from his wardrobe, it probably will not go well with the trousers etc. Many times I have been embarrassed to see him using a dark grey handkerchief which should have been white. Funnily he does not seem to miss colour as much as he did at the outset of his problem. He seldom asks about the colour of the countryside or flowers, etc., and seems to have accepted the limitations of living in a black-and-white world.

However, if you ask John what is his most difficult problem, he will say visual agnosia. That inability to recognise me or friends or where he is causes more frustration than anything else. It does mean that I have to rely on friends and family to look after him if I am not around. Luckily we have friends who understand John's problem but still find pleasure in his company as he can contribute interesting tales and facts from his long-term memory. One friend in particular, Dennis by name, has taken us on several outings to include museums of World War II. Dennis is able to describe tanks, guns, aeroplanes, the Overlord Tapestry, etc. in detail and in a technical language which John understands. John adds his comments and thoroughly enjoys such visits even if he is largely seeing through another's eyes. Kind Dennis made a model of the Lysander aircraft which John once flew and John delights in explaining its detail to any visitor who notices it flying from the lounge ceiling. However, on these excursions, it is Dennis's wife, Muriel, who makes sure John does not trip over awkward steps or drinks his wine and not someone else's at lunch.

The thousands of people who look after handicapped people will understand how important friends are not only to the handicapped but to those responsible for their care. I relax totally when the family or friends are around to amuse or care for John and when we go to Birmingham to visit Professor Humphreys and Professor Riddoch, I enjoy handing over the patient and going off to spend a few hours in the shops. To John, any help he can give the scientists in their research remains his greatest pleasure. To all those clever men and women we have met over the years I can only say 'It was an honour to know you and thank you for all your help.' The friendship we have been given, and the understanding of our problems prove how much help medical people can give their patients. One realises what busy people they are and, if in return for the hours they have spent with us, John and his handler are delighted to make a contribution to their research. You may wonder why the handler is included but one has to remember he has to be taken to all appointments!

John's answer

Five years on and frustration is still my hated driver. To feel so near visual comprehension and endlessly to find myself in error or incomprehension comes as a biting stab but also, like a spur, a goad to another effort. Having notched my three score and ten, I accept a natural slowing as normal, but where I should be mellow and more accepting of men's faults and follies, I am unforgivingly critical that they should waste or disuse their normal abilities and gifts. I accept that this must be the result of an innate jealousy and a strong 'Poor Me' syndrome – but it is so!

My problems are still as acute as ever. Only last week I lost my way home from the local post office though I had insisted I was fully confident to do the journey solo. I lost my way on the return journey of about 750 metres, which I have taken while accompanied every week for the last six years. The fact that I ended up in the local off licence (where wine and liquor can be bought) was fortuitous, but made Iris deeply suspicious.

Life after Iris

Iris was diagnosed with stomach cancer in 1990 and died in 1991. John moved into a semi-sheltered home where he could look after himself generally in his room, but took meals with other residents who were able to make sure he ate only the correct food! His first floor room had a bay window which overlooked a shaded courtyard. He was able to fit two armchairs and small table into the bay, and this was a pleasant spot in which to entertain his visitors. His son's family lived almost directly opposite the home on the other side of the road, and there was a tree at their gateway which served as a useful identifying landmark. The home itself had a lovely garden, filled with roses in the summer. John made friends with the gardener, and was able, under strict guidance, to carry out gardening duties. For most of the time John was there, the other residents were women. Lunch was the main meal of the day and they would all gather around a large table. John was asked how he could tell who was who when they were all seated and he replied:

> Ah, I have all my ladies so that I know their voices, so I can be as polite as hell by saying, 'Good morning girls' – that is very important, and they say, 'Good morning, John'. Now, I therefore have only got to recognise about eight sounds and that's not difficult when you hear it every day. You can pin eight sounds to eight girls but, in order to make quite sure, a little habit you may have realised: I call all girls 'dear' – the whole damn lot because they can't find me wanting! At my age, you can say 'dear' and nobody will take offence.

After moving to his new residence, John was given as 'homework' a series of written questions, and asked to write the answers. These are listed below:

How do you orient yourself in a new environment (e.g., imagine you have been invited to drinks in a home you have not visited before), how do you manage?
Usually very badly when after daylight has gone and/or curtains are drawn. A fireplace is usually the social centre of a room but flats and modern designed houses often don't have such.

Give examples of problems you have encountered in a new environment.
My main difficulties are caused by my poor 3D visual state. A brick on the pavement may be only a piece of paper. A hole in the floor or a small step up or down often look the same. A slope on the floor (as often in large shops) has bad results to my walking.

How do you recognise the other residents?
My problem is explained to them all. Therefore, they are asked to say something in view of me to aid my problem. When food and drink are served at table, I am told what is on offer. My family have to do this when we go out for a meal.

How do you manage meals, and how do you distinguish edible from inedible (e.g., a lemon slice) items on your plate?

Quite simply, I never eat alone. I always have to eat where family or friends who know my problems are close to tell me what and where items are on my plate. Exceptions are very obvious: like boiled eggs, bananas, etc. but not mixed vegetables or meats, except the obvious, such as sausages.

Over the years since you have had agnosia, do you think your recognition of anything has improved? Give examples where this improvement is shown.

I really do not think it has improved. I believe my sense of background, size and relationship to background are still my only skills of recognition. For some reason, moving objects are always easier to recognise. Moving my head to give my brains extra viewpoints is my normal reaction.

Over the years since you have had agnosia, do you think your recognition of anything has got worse?

No, rather the opposite. Since childhood I was taught by my school masters to use my logic to explain things or ideas not understood. As my parents lived overseas I had little contact with any alternatives or other ideas. Service in the forces both pre-war and World War II widened my general education considerably and much strengthened my belief in early marriage to an intelligent partner, who had learning and skills in matters I had never even heard of.

How well do you remember what different animals or objects look like?

I am daily conscious of how my memory of plants, shrubs and flowers has deteriorated especially as gardening and general horticulture have always been one of my main interests and hobbies.

Can you remember the colours of different objects and animals?

No, I cannot. Logic tells that a rose bush in flower has bright colours but I can only guess what are petals and what are leaves by the light they reflect. Just like an old black-and-white camera picture.

Do you dream? Are the dreams in colour?

Yes, I do; even from ill-remembered early childhood, I have dreamed nightly and in both fanciful and illogical dreams, and most days a type of shallow, fancy, awakening time dreams which I know at the time are only dreams. But colour, alas, I think not.

Has your reading improved? Can you now read your own writing?

I try to mentally prepare my next few words and then write by 'short memory' as it were, before I forget what I have in mind to say. If I do this, I can recognise some words but otherwise it remains as difficult as ever. If I am interrupted, I often cannot read my last sentence.

Do you recognise yourself now in a mirror?

Only by logical thought. Because of lifetime practice, I can shave in the dark by touch alone so I do not encounter myself then. However, there are times when I have stepped aside from the mirror to let someone else pass – only to realise it must have been me.

How do you manage to coordinate the colours of your clothes (socks, tie, shirt)?

Left alone, I do very badly. Look at any old black-and-white photo of people. How can you tell the colour of their clothes?

Do you watch television? What strategies do you use?

I watch a lot of television because I avoid the strain and impossibility of reading any print. What I find hardest is that used on computers, and similar visual equipment.

How do you know which number to ring when telephoning people?

I have a receiver rest equipped with 12 very large numbers and letters. I answer my phone using one of four languages. This works wonderfully.

Testing visual recognition over time

Our own impressions of whether our recognition changes over time, and why we might sometimes succeed and sometimes fail, are not necessarily accurate. John wrote that his sense of background was one of the things he relies on, but the evidence suggests a more subtle point. John was abnormally poor when required to segment the background and fore-ground parts of an image from two-dimensional cues alone (see Chapter 6). Where he succeeded was under the particular conditions where he could use either movement or depth to help him form a sense of back-ground. His use of this information was something that improved over time, indexed by an increased ability to recognise real objects, but John was not aware of why it improved.

We formally assessed John's visual recognition abilities at 14 and 16 years after his stroke (in 1995 and 1997) [99]. Figure 11.1 presents John's copies of line drawings. John was at least as accurate at copying line drawings in 1997 as he was in 1982. Interestingly, he remained unable to identify any of the exemplars shown in the figure.

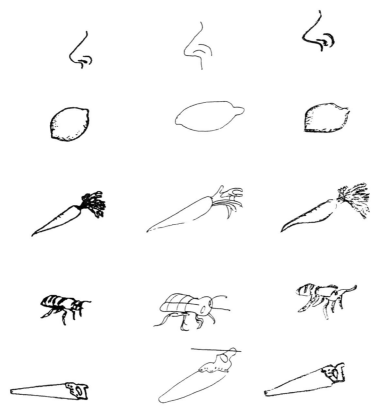

Figure 11.1 Example of John's copying. Left: exemplar line drawings that he was asked to copy. Centre: copies carried out in 1982. Right: copies made in 1997.

Source: From Riddoch, M. J. *et al.* (1999). Memories are made of this: the effects of time on stored visual knowledge in a case of visual agnosia. *Brain* 122: 537–559, by permission of Oxford University Press.

When John's identification of objects was examined, we found that there was some improvement in his naming of real objects – with about 20 per cent more objects named in 1997 compared with 1982. His naming of line drawings remained at the same level, however, with the exception of some improvement in the identification of tools. In Chapter 9, we noted that John was better able to name objects that had strong 'affordances', measured by whether the objects evoked a response based on the position of their handle. It is possible that the improved naming of tools reflected some sensitisation to these action-related properties of the stimuli. John remained abnormally affected by presenting the stimuli for short durations and if drawings were overlapping. Our conclusion was that the fundamental perceptual deficit underlying John's agnosia remained much the same, but that he had learned to capitalise on the visual cues remaining available to him (e.g., depth information which aided the recognition of real objects) and to action-related cues for objects he interacted with (e.g, tools).

We also evaluated John's memory for objects. Note that, in his own descriptions, John reported that his memory for objects had deteriorated. We were able to confirm this in tests of drawing from memory. Figure 11.2 shows examples of John's drawing from memory in 1985 and 1995 (he was asked to draw an owl and celery on each occasion). In the early years after his lesion, as we have noted, John showed accurate drawing from memory for objects he could no longer recognise. However, over the subsequent years, his drawings deteriorated and showed a kind of regression towards more general forms for animals, fruits and vegetables especially. It was as if he was losing the specific details that characterised individual animals, fruits and vegetables, and was left only with those properties that held across the whole of that class of objects.

The difficulties John had in drawing from memory were not just due to him having to draw; nor did they reflect some general deterioration in memory. Note that John's drawing remained good when he was asked to copy objects (Figure 11.1). General memory was tested by asking him to give verbal definitions of objects from memory. There was a striking contrast between definitions taken in 1985 and in 1995. Whereas his definitions in 1985 often contained impressive detail about the visual properties of objects, in 1995 he reported considerable detail about the history of the objects, what actions were performed with the objects, where they might be found etc., but less information was provided about what objects looked like. An example is given in Figure 11.3. We counted up the number of visual and verbal attributes of objects that John spontaneously produced in his definitions. Across the years between the

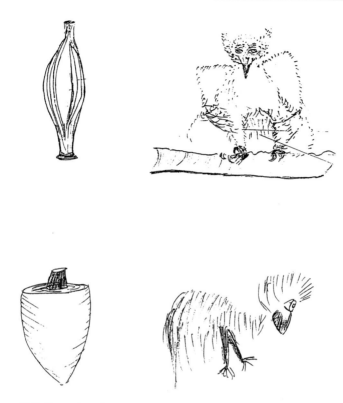

Figure 11.2 Examples of John's drawings from memory in 1985 (top) and 1995 (bottom). Left: celery. Right: an owl.

Source: From Riddoch, M. J. *et al.* (1999). Memories are made of this: the effects of time on stored visual knowledge in a case of visual agnosia. *Brain* 122: 537–559, by permission of Oxford University Press.

initial and subsequent tests, John produced fewer visual attributes (there were about 10 per cent fewer attributes listed in 1995 than in 1985) and more 'verbal' attributes (his listing of verbal attributes increased by about 20 per cent). Thus, there was not an overall deterioration in John's memory as he grew older, but there was a selective shift in the things he could and could not remember. Memory for verbal and functional attributes did not decrease, whereas his memory for visual detail did.

This evidence for a selective loss of visual knowledge has subsequently been replicated in other longer-term follow-ups of agnosic

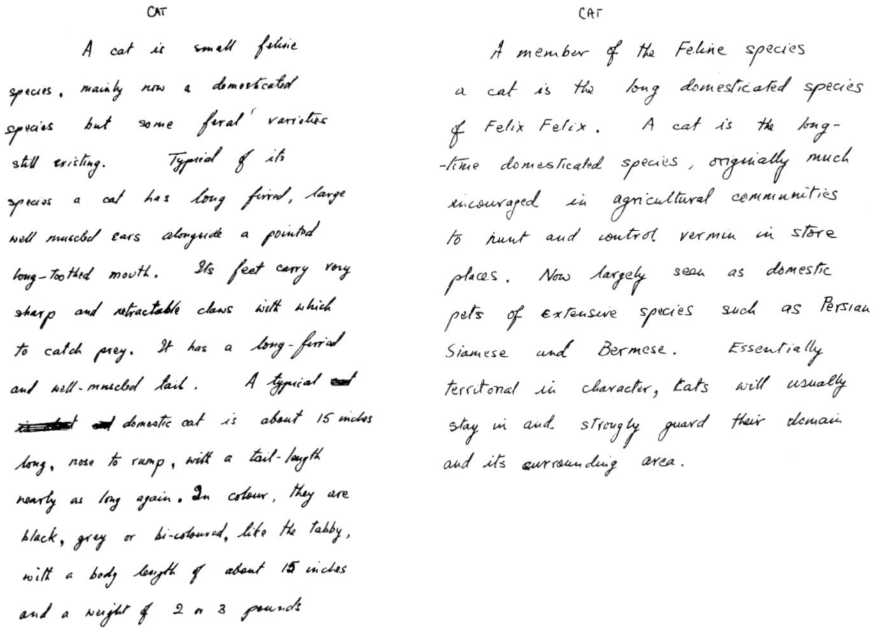

CAT

A member of the Feline species
a cat is the long domesticated species
of Felix Felix. A cat is the long-
-time domesticated species, originally much
encouraged in agricultural communities
to hunt and control vermin in store
places. Now largely seen as domestic
pets of extensive species such as Persian
Siamese and Burmese. Essentially
territorial in character, cats will usually
stay in and strongly guard their domain
and its surrounding area.

CAT

A cat is small feline
species, mainly new & domesticated
species but some feral varieties
still existing. Typical of its
genus a cat has long furred, large
well muscled ears alongside a pointed
long-farted mouth. Its feet carry very
sharp and retractable claws with which
to catch prey. It has a long-furred
and well-muscled tail. A typical
domestic cat is about 15 inches
long, nose to rump, with a tail length
nearly as long again. In colour, they are
black, grey or bi-coloured, like the Tabby,
with a body length of about 15 inches
and a weight of 2 n 3 pounds.

Figure 11.3 Examples of John's verbal definitions of a cat in 1985 and 1995

Source: From Riddoch, M. J. et al. (1999). Memories are made of this: the effects of time on stored visual knowledge in a case of visual agnosia. *Brain* 122: 537–559, by permission of Oxford University Press.

patients. For example, in another agnosic patient we worked with, DW, there was a striking similarity to the data from John [100]. Just like John, DW's drawings from memory deteriorated over time though his copying abilities remained the same. Just like John, DW's definitions of objects from memory contained fewer visual and more verbal/functional attributes when he was re-tested after 12 years. In both DW and John, the decrease in reporting specific visual attributes of objects was most pronounced for animals, fruits and vegetables, perhaps because these stimuli tend to have more similar structures which can regress back to a common but undifferentiated prototype when not consistently upgraded.

To account for these results, we suggest that our visual knowledge of the world is not static, stored away like a book on a library shelf. Rather this knowledge is dynamically updated ('re-calibrated') as we interact with the world. This re-calibration process does not operate at very early stages of vision, however, which were spared in John. Rather the calibration process operates on 'intermediate' visual representations – where elements are integrated into detailed descriptions of objects parts in relation to the perceptual whole. Where these intermediate representations are disrupted, as was the case for John, then re-calibration does not take place, with the result being that precise visual knowledge about objects deteriorates.

The close parallel between the loss of visual knowledge in patients such as John and their recognition impairment suggests that visual perception and visual memory/mental imagery are closely linked processes – a conclusion we also made from our analysis of John's perception and memory for faces (Chapter 8). It appears that, at least when we want to remember/imagine visual detail, we need to re-activate processes also required to visually recognise the same stimulus. Damage to these processes degrades both perception and imagery.

Rehabilitation

The changes we have noted in John's object processing over time were not linked to any specific training programme. We can ask, though, whether his recognition would have improved if he had been given targeted training. Clearly this question is difficult to answer in the absence of a consistent learning programme. However, the attempts we made to retrain John's perception met with only limited success. In Chapter 6, we noted the experiments where John was given extensive practice (over 3000 learning trials) at grouping simple visual stimuli (Ts in different orientations) in order to segment the target from groups of distractors.

Despite multiple sessions of practice, we were not able to make John's search efficient and there remained abnormally strong effects of the number of elements present. Training John to group visual elements was not successful.

What about retraining his object recognition? In one small-scale study, we had John learn a set of six line drawings and six faces of famous people [101]. One week after the second of two learning sessions we tested him on (1) exactly the same stimuli he had been trained on; (2) pictures of the same stimuli but from a slightly different point of view (typically a shift of ~45 degree of angle in depth); and (3) a set of items that he had not been trained on that were matched in complexity to the trained stimuli. We also examined his naming of new line drawings of objects from the category he had been trained on (e.g., an Alsatian dog when a Labrador was in the original training set). John retained his learning of the repeated images and re-identified all these items correctly. However, there was relatively little generalisation of this learning to either the same objects shown from a different view or to different items from the same category (from one dog to another; for example, having learned to name a Labrador as a dog, he then named the Alsatian as a horse). These, admittedly small-scale, studies suggest that the generalisation of perceptual learning (perhaps like the updating of long-term visual memory) depends on having good intermediate-level visual processes that can be commonly accessed by the same objects when seen from different viewpoints and by different objects with similar perceptual structures (different exemplars of the same basic object). With damage to these processes visual learning can still take place, but it is constrained to operate on representations that are 'image-based' and non-optimal for perceptual generalisation.

Conclusion

Our re-testing of John indicated that the perceptual state of an individual is not static but changes over time, according to the visual experiences we have and the processes available to keep our perceptual systems calibrated to the world. Processes that are preserved after a lesion – in John's case, the analysis of stereoscopic depth and action-based inter-actions with objects – may come to be weighted more heavily in a patient's perceptual decisions, and processes not upgraded (precise visual knowledge about objects) may degrade. The data also indicate that the updating of long-term visual memory, and the generalisation of learn-ing across different views and objects, depend on intermediate-level processes of grouping and segmentation, and both the updating process and new learning can be limited when these processes are impaired. However, it should be recognised that our understanding of brain plasticity and how to enhance functional recovery after a brain lesion has still a long way to go, and developments such a direct brain stimulation, which are now being explored, were not available at the time John had his lesion. We very much look forward to the systematic exploration of ways to stimulate functional recovery in patients, which can be applied to help individuals such as John in the future.

We can close, though, with the parting words that Iris wrote to close the original *To See But Not To See* [87],which summarise well the journey made by John and Iris after his fateful appendectomy.

Writing about their experience of five years, Iris stated:

We have now worked out a happy partnership with both of us accepting what we can and cannot do. John does some dusting and vacuum cleaning fairly well, but as he tends to dust some items twice and others not at all, I take over when visitors are expected. He opens the garage door, carries the shopping, posts letters, makes the tea and as long as I leave the bottle in the right place, pours himself a glass of sherry. When we have guests, I have to pour the drinks otherwise they may not get what they expect!

If there is a beautiful sunset, I try and paint a word picture for him so he can join in my pleasure. Similarly I have to describe floral arrangements and the colour of the shirt and tie I have selected for him to wear. This colour problem creates difficulties as, if I relax my vigilance, he uses a dirty white handkerchief or wears odd socks, but his sense of touch has improved so that socks are no longer inside out. I still question his reasoning power. For example, he saw a dog swimming in a river and asked if it was a swan – had he said an otter, I would not have been surprised. He has sometimes taken my rain-coat from the cupboard instead of his own, not apparently working out that the buttons were on the wrong side. Possibly such lapses are due to lack of concentration as I know he has to think what he is doing all the time. When taking the rubbish to the dustbin, a job I do without thinking, he has to say to himself 'left outside the front door'. Although he leaves business matters to me, he likes to know about them so all letters are read to him and he makes comments and suggestions. His dependence on me to take him for walks, to drive the car, tell him what clothes to wear, arrange our daily programme, etc., must be very frustrating to him. I admit it is a harder job than

I had expected to do in my old age, but it has its compensations. Had things been different I should never have met some very interesting, kind, caring and clever medical and scientific people, who have given me great support, help and friendship. Neither should I have had the opportunity of seeing some fascinating machines in operation or watching research workers at work.

We are lucky to have family and friends with whom we exchange visits. We try and avoid parties as John does not like crowded rooms where noise prevents him hearing other people's voices and he has to ask me to steer him towards people to whom he wishes to speak. At meals he is always seated next to a kind person who can stop him eating the shells of prawns, the lemon at the side of the fish or putting salt instead of sugar on his strawberries. It is to his credit that, in spite of his problem, he has always remained his cheerful self, never moaning, and if he sometimes loses his temper, then, who wouldn't?

Chapter 12

Obituary[1]

John (1921–2008)[2]

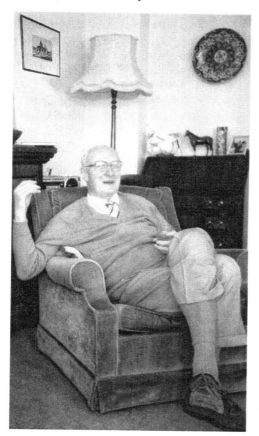

Figure 12.1 John enjoying a glass of sherry. On the wall to his left is the etching of St Paul's Cathedral, which he was asked to draw (see Chapter 3, Figure 3.2).

Source: Reprinted from G. Humphreys and Riddoch, M. J. (2008) John (1921–2008). *Cortex* 44: 759–761, with permission from Elsevier.

Patients are the unsung heroes of neuropsychology. John was an unsung hero of numerous neuropsychological tests over 26 years after suffering a stroke in 1981. The stroke resulted in damage to posterior ventral cortex, with a magnetic resonance imaging (MRI) scan in 2006 revealing damage from areas V2–V3 through the lingual and fusiform gyri into the temporal lobe. Following this stroke, John presented with several neuropsychological problems, most notably visual agnosia, but also prosopagnosia, alexia without agraphia, achromatopsia and topographical agnosia. A case report and book, both published in 1987 [56, 94], established him as the classic case of 'integrative agnosia', with his object recognition attributed to a deficit in intermediate visual processes concerned with the integration of part elements into whole shapes, particularly under conditions in which there are complex figure–ground relations between the elements in an image. Despite this perceptual deficit, John was able to reproduce line drawings in a highly accurate fashion. This led to a revision of the long-standing dichotomy between 'apperceptive' and 'associative' agnosia, based on the simple clinical diagnostic of whether the patient could copy objects that they could not identify.

In John's case, there was good copying, but still an underlying perceptual locus to his agnosia. In subsequent work it was demonstrated that the processes involved in computing edges from oriented elements were spared [59], providing evidence for a separation between the computation of edges and the organisation of edges into shapes. This problem in organising the relations between elements in shapes also dissociated from the ability to average across edge orientations, aspects of which were also retained [60]. There were also dissociations between the processing of form and the ability to use depth information. Like many agnosic patients, John was better at identifying real objects than line drawings. In his case this could be traced back to his use of binocular and motion disparity cues to 'parse' objects into appropriate surfaces [78]. When dealing with faces, John's perception showed a breakdown in processing configural information, showing superiority in dealing with face parts compared with wholes [71]. Despite this, he was able to derive information from facial emotions using partonomic cues [73], providing evidence for partonomic information being used in coding facial emotions. In addition, he showed a good ability to use motion cues for emotion judgements [74]. Thus, the ability to use motion dissociated from the impaired processing of static form information. Meeting him in everyday life, you would not notice that he had any problem in face processing, and he responded appropriately in social interactions.

John's deficit in form processing was profound and there was no evidence for implicit access to knowledge of objects [66]. In contrast to this, there was evidence for residual processing of colour, despite a clear inability to make conscious colour judgement [77]. The studies of John's colour processing suggested that there could be some colour processing using a parallel residual pathway distinct from the parvocellular pathway normally supporting colour perception (and damaged in his case).

John's pronounced problems in processing visual forms sat alongside a hugely impressive store of knowledge about objects, and as testers it was our continued delight to receive his highly articulate descriptions and his detailed drawings of objects from long-term memory. However, in repeated testing across the years, it was possible to observe deterioration in his detailed visual knowledge about objects, while his verbal knowledge remained at a level that continued to out-shine our students. Similarly, John's visual knowledge about faces was good until tests probed the representation of configural knowledge that he also found difficult to perceive [76]. These results point to important interactions between perception and memory, with intact visual processing serving to keep visual memory accurately calibrated [91]. Studies of John's visual short-term memory also revealed a close parallel between the visual elements that he was impaired at perceiving and the information that he found difficult to retain [82]. The data here suggested that visual short-term memory is contingent on representations also used in on-line visual perception.

As all who conducted research with John will attest, he was a dedicated participant and a highly reliable observer. He would work throughout a day within minimal breaks, with only the promise of a dry sherry as a reward. He enjoyed meeting many researchers from across the world and never failed to respond with anything other than patience and perseverance, despite the occasionally odd or unclear instructions! We could recount many anecdotes. The first time we tested John it poured with rain and Jane slipped into a puddle at the bottom of the stairs leading to the house where he and his wife lived. Jane then ended up testing John in his wife's dressing gown! To compound things further the testing involved John identifying objects by touch with Jane passing the stimuli from under dining room table – his wife was not greatly impressed! There was also a lovely moment during the making of a film for the BBC when the director thought it would be fun to have John wait in a line for a taxi and placed his wife before him in the line. John, giving a running commentary, revealed his concern that the woman next in line seemed to be over-familiar with him! Then glancing down, he recognised his wife from her ankles and shoes! On another occasion a customer at a checkout was amazed to find him packing her bags and taking the shopping out, with John having the mistaken belief that she was his wife! John died after a short illness in January 2008. He will be missed as a rare 'rabbit' (his words) for science, and, on a personal level, as a friend over many years.

Notes

1   Reprinted from G. Humphreys and M. J. Riddoch (2008) 'John (1921–2008)', *Cortex*, 44: 759–761, with permission from Elsevier.
2   In our scientific papers John was known as John, which were his initials, although he was always known by his middle name, John.

Bibliography

[1] Warrington, E. K. and Taylor, A. Two categorical stages of object recognition. *Perception* **9**, 152–164 (1978).

[2] Hubel, D. H. and Wiesel, T. N. Receptive fields of single neurones: the cat's visual cortex. *Journal of Physiology (London)* **160**, 106–154 (1959).

[3] Van Essen, D. C. *et al.* Mapping visual cortex in monkeys and humans using surface-based atlases. *Vision Research* **41**, 1359–1378 (2001).

[4] Zeki, S. M. Functional specialisation in the visual cortex of the rhesus monkey. *Nature* **274**, 423–428 (1978).

[5] Sakata, H. *et al.* Neural coding of 3D features of objects for hand action in the parietal cortex of the monkey. *Philosophical Transactions of the Royal Society, London, Series B*, 1363–1373 (1998).

[6] Ungerleider, L. G. and Mishkin, M. Two cortical visual systems. In *Analysis of Visual Behavior* (eds J. Ingle, M. A. Goodale, and R. J. W. Mansfield) pp. 549–586 (Cambridge, MA: MIT Press, 1982).

[7] Gazzaniga, M. S., Ivry, R. B. and Mangun, G. R. *Cognitve Neuroscience* (New York: W. W. Norton and Co., 1998).

[8] Zeki, S. *et al.* A direct demonstration of functional specialisation in human visual cortex. *Journal of Neuroscience* **11**, 641–649 (1991).

[9] Hebb, D. O. *The Organization of Behaviour* (Chichester: John Wiley and Sons, 1949).

[10] Bruce, C., Desimone, R. and Gross, C. G. Visual properties of neurons in a polysensory area in superior temporal sulcus of the macaque. *Journal of Neurophysiology* **46**, 369–384 (1981).

[11] Von der Heydt, R., Peterhans, E. and Baumgartner, G. Illursory contours and cortical neuron responses. *Science* **224**, 1260–1262 (1984).

[12] Lee, T. S. and Nguyen, M. Dynamics of subjective contour formation in the early visual cortex. *Proceedings of the National Academy of Sciences of the United States of America* **98**, 1907–1911 (2001).

[13] Maertens, M., Pollmann, S., Hanke, M., Mildner, T. and Möller, H. Retinotopic activation in response to subjective contours in primary visual cortex. *Frontiers in Human Neuroscience* **2**, 1–6 (2008).

[14] Singer, W. and Gray, C. M. Visual feature integration and the temporal correlation hypothesis. *Annual Review of Neuroscience* **18**, 555–586 (1995).

[15] Schwarzkopf, D. S. and Kourtzi, Z. Experience shapes the utility of natural statistics for perceptual contour integration. *Current Biology* **18**, 1162–1167 (2008).

[16] Navon, D. Forest before trees: the precedence of global features in visual perception. *Cognitive Psychology* **9**, 353–383 (1977).

[17] Tanaka, K., Saito, H. A., Fukada, Y. and Moriya, M. Coding visual images of objects in the infero-temporal cortex of the macaque monkey. *Journal of Neurophysiology* **66**, 170–189 (1991).

[18] Perrett, D. I., Hietanen, J. K., Oram, M. W. and Benson, P. J. Organization and functions of cells responsive to faces in the temporal cortex. *Philosophical Transactions of the Royal Society of London Series B – Biological Sciences* **335**, 23–30 (1992).

[19] Gross, C. G., Rocha-Miranda, C. E. and Bender, D. B. Visual properties of neurons in inferotemporal cortex of macaque. *Journal of Neurophysiology* **35**, 96–111 (1972).

[20] Vuilleumier, P., Henson, R. N., Driver, J. and Dolan, R. J. Multiple levels of visual object constancy revealed by event-related fMRI of repetition priming. *Nature Neuroscience* **5**, 491–499 (2002).

[21] Kourtzi, Z. and Kanwisher, N. Cortical regions involved in perceiving object shape. *Journal of Neuroscience* **20**, 3310–3318 (2000).

[22] James, T. W. *et al.* Haptic study of three-dimensional objects activates extrastriate visual areas. *Neuropsychologia* **40**, 1706–1714 (2002).

[23] Roberts, K. L. and Humphreys, G. W. Action relationships concatenate representations of separate objects in the ventral visual system. *Neuroimage* **52**, 1541–1548 (2010).

[24] Goh, J. O. S. *et al.* Cortical areas involved in object, background, and object background processing revealed with functional magnetic resonance adaptation. *Journal of Neuroscience* **24**, 10223–10228 (2004).

[25] Motter, B. C. Neural correlates of feature selective memory and pop-out in extrastriate area V4. *Journal of Neuroscience* **14**, 2190–2199 (1994).

[26] Schneider, K. A. and Kastner, S. Effects of sustained spatial attention in the human lateral geniculate nucleus and superior colliculus. *Journal of Neuroscience* **29**, 1784–1795 (2009).

[27] Courtney, S. M., Ungeleider, L. G., Keil, K. and Haxby, J. V. Object and spatial visual working memory activate separate neural systems in human cortex. *Cerebral Cortex* **6**, 39–49 (1996).

[28] Berryhill, M. E. and Olson, I. R. The representation of object distance: evidence from neuroimaging and neuropsychology. *Frontiers in Human Neuroscience* **3** (2009).

[29] Culham, J. C. *et al.* Visually guided grasping produces fMRI activation in dorsal but not ventral stream brain areas. *Experimental Brain Research* **153**, 180–189 (2003).

[30] Thompson, P. Margaret Thatcher: a new illusion. *Perception* **9**, 483–484 (1980).

[31] Takane, Y. and Sergent, J. Multidimensional scaling models for reaction times and same–different judgements. *Psychometrika* **48**, 393–423 (1983).

[32] Liu, J., Harris, A. and Kanwisher, N. Stages of processing in face perception: an MEG study. *Nature Neuroscience* **5**, 910–916 (2002).

[33] Pitcher, D., Dilks, D. D., Saxe, R. R., Triantafyllou, C. and Kanwisher, N. Differential selectivity for dynamic versus static information in face-selective cortical regions. *Neuroimage* **56**, 2356–2363 (2011).

[34] Gauthier, I., Tarr, M. J., Andersen, R. A., Skudlarski, P. and Gore, J. Activation in the middle fusiform 'face area' increases with expertise in recognising novel objects. *Nature Neuroscience* **2**, 568–573 (1999).

[35] Vinckier, F. *et al.* Hierarchical coding of letter strings in the ventral stream: dissecting the inner organization of the visual word-form system. *Neuron* **55**, 143–156 (2007).

[36] Dehaene, S. and Cohen, L. The unique role of the visual word form area in reading. *Trends in Cognitive Sciences* **15**, 254–262 (2011).

[37] Dehaene, S. *et al.* How learning to read changes the cortical networks for vision and language. *Science* **330**, 1359–1364 (2010).

[38] Macrae, D. and Trolle, E. The defect in function in visual agnosia. *Brain* **79**, 94–110 (1956).

[39] Munk, H. *Ueber die Funktionen der Grosshirnrinde* (Hirschwald, 1881).

[40] Lissauer, H. Ein Fall von Seelenblindheit nebst einem Beitrage zur Theorie derselben. *Archiv für Psychiatrie und Nervenkrankheiten* **21**, 222–270 (1890).

[41] Wilbrand, H. *Die Seelenblindheit als Herderscheinung und ihre Beziehungen zur homonymen Hemianopsie, zur Alexie und zur Agraphie* (Bergmann, 1887).

[42] Freund, C. S. Über optische Aphasie und Seelenblindheit. *Archiv für Psychiatrie und Nervenkrankheiten* **20**, 371–416 (1889).

[43] Bender, M. B. and Feldman, M. The so-called 'visual agnosias'. *Brain* **9**, 173–186 (1972).

[44] Critchley, M. The problem of visual agnosia. *Journal of Neurological Science* **1**, 274–290 (1964).

[45] Bay, E. Disturbances of visual perception and their examination. *Brain* **76**, 515–551 (1953).

[46] Ettlinger, G., Warrington, E. and Zangwill, O. L. A further study of visual-spatial agnosia. *Brain* **80**, 335–361 (1957).

[47] Ettlinger, G. and Wyke, M. Deficits in identifying objects visually in a patient with cerebrovascular disease. *Journal of Neurology, Neurosurgery & Psychiatry* **24**, 254–259 (1961).

[48] Cowey, A. and Weiskrantz, L. A comparison of the effects of inferotemporal and striate cortex lesions on the visual behaviour of rhesus monkeys. *The Quarterly Journal of Experimental Psychology* **19**, 246–253 (1967).

[49] Semmes, J. Agnosia in animals and man. *Psychological Review* **60**, 140–147 (1953).

[50] Riddoch, M. J. and Humphreys, G. W. Visual object processing in optic aphasia: a case of semantic access agnosia. *Cognitive Neuropsychology* **4**, 131–185 (1987).

[51] Fery, P. and Morais, J. A case study of visual agnosia without perceptual processing or structural descriptions impairment. *Cognitive Neuropsychology* **20**, 595–618 (2003).

[52] Humphreys, G. W. and Forde, E. M. E. Naming a giraffe but not an animal: base-level but not superordinate naming in a patient with impaired semantics. *Cognitive Neuropsychology* **22**, 539–558 (2005).

[53] Efron, R. What is perception? *Boston Studies in Philosophy of Science* **4**, 137–173 (1968).

[54] Benson, D. F. and Greenberg, J. P. Visual form agnosia: a specific deficit in visual discrimination. *Archives of Neurology* **20**, 82–89 (1969).

[55] Milner, A. D. *et al.* Perception and action in 'visual form agnosia'. *Brain* **114**, 405–428 (1991).

[56] Campion, J. and Latto, R. Apperceptive agnosia due to carbon monoxide poisoning: an interpretation based on critical band masking from disseminated lesions. *Behavioural Brain Research* **15**, 227–240 (1985).

[57] Warrington, E. K. Constructional apraxia. In *Handbook of Clinical Neurology*, vol. 45 (eds P. J. Vinken, G. W. Bruyn, and H. L. Klawans) (Oxford: Elsevier Science Publishers, 1985).

[58] Riddoch, M. J. and Humphreys, G. W. A case of integrative agnosia. *Brain* **110**, 1431–1462 (1987).

[59] Humphreys, G. W., Riddoch, M. J., Quinlan, P. T., Donnelly, N. and Price, C. A. Parallel pattern processing and visual agnosia. *Canadian Journal of Psychology* **46**, 377–416 (1992).

[60] Humphreys, G. W. and Riddoch, M. J. Routes to object constancy: implications from neurological impairments of object constancy. *Quarterly Journal of Experimental Psychology* **36A**, 385–415 (1984).

[61] Giersch, A., Humphreys, G. W., Boucart, M. and Kovátks, I. The computation of occluded contours in visual agnosia: evidence of early computation prior to shape binding and figure-ground coding. *Cognitive Neuropsychology* **17**, 731–759 (2000).

[62] Allen, H. A., Humphreys, G. W. and Bridge, H. Ventral extra-striate cortical areas are required for optimal orientation averaging. *Vision Research* **47**, 766–775 (2007).

[63] Geschwind, N. Disconnection syndromes in animals and man. *Brain* **88**, 237–294, 585–644 (1965).

[64] Riddoch, M. J. *et al.* A tale of two agnosias: distinctions between form and integrative agnosia. *Cognitive Neuropsychology* **25**, 56–92 (2008).

[65] Riddoch, M. J. and Humphreys, G. W. Object identification in simultanagnosia: when wholes are not the sum of their parts. *Cognitive Neuropsychology* **21**, 423–441 (2004).

[66] Lawson, R. and Humphreys, G. W. The effects of view in depth on the identification of line drawings and silhouettes of familiar objects: normality and pathology. *Visual Cognition* **6**, 165–195 (1999).

[67] Humphreys, G. W., Riddoch, M. J. and Quinlan, P. T. Interactive processes in perceptual organization: evidence from visual agnosia. In *Attention and Performance XI* (eds M. I. Posner and O. S. M. Marin) (Hillsdale, NJ: Erlbaum, 1985).

[68] Hubel, D. H. and Livingstone, M. S. Segregation of form, color, and stereopsis in primate area 18. *Journal of Neuroscience* **7**, 3378–3415 (1987).

[69] Boucart, M. and Humphreys, G. W. The computation of perceptual structure from collinearity and closure: normality and pathology. *Neuropsychologia* **30**, 527–546 (1992).

[70] Boucart, M. and Humphreys, G. W. Global shape cannot be attended without object identification. *Journal of Experimental Psychology: Human Perception and Performance* **18**, 785–806 (1992).

[71] Mevorach, C., Humphreys, G. W. and Shalev, L. Attending to local form while ignoring global aspects depends on handedness: evidence from TMS. *Nature Neuroscience* **8**, 276–277 (2005).

[72] Riddoch, M. J., Johnston, R. A., Bracewell, R. M., Boutsen, L. and Humphreys, G. W. Are faces special? A case of pure prosopagnosia. *Cognitive Neuropsychology* **25**, 3–26 (2008).

[73] Boutsen, L. and Humphreys, G. W. Face context interferes with local part processing in a prosopagnosic patient. *Neuropsychologia* **40**, 2305–2313 (2002).

[74] De Gelder, B. and Rouw, R. Paradoxical configuration effects for faces and objects in prosopagnosia. *Neuropsychologia* **38**, 1271–1279 (2000).

[75] Baudouin, J.-Y. and Humphreys, G. W. Compensatory strategies in processing facial emotions: evidence from prosopagnosia. *Neuropsychologia* **44**, 1361–1369 (2006).

[76] Humphreys, G. W., Donnelly, N. and Riddoch, M. J. Expression is computed separately from facial identity and it is computed separately for moving and static faces: neuropsychological evidence. *Neuropsychologia* **31**, 173–181 (1993).

[77] Lander, K., Humphreys, G. and Bruce, V. Exploring the role of motion in prosopagnosia: recognizing, learning and matching faces. *Neurocase* **10**, 462–470 (2004).

[78] Young, A. W., Humphreys, G. W., Riddoch, M. J., Hellawell, D. J. and De Haans, E. H. F. Recognition impairments and face imagery. *Neuropsychologia* **32**, 693–702 (1994).

[79] De Haan, E. H. F., Young, A. W. and Newcombe, F. Face recognition without awareness. *Cognitive Neuropsychology* **4**, 385–415 (1987).

[80] Humphreys, G. W. *et al.* Face recognition and awareness after brain injury. In *The Neuropsychology of Consciousness.* (eds A. D. Milner and M. D. Rugg) (New York: Academic Press, 1992).

[81] Troscianko, T. *et al.* Human colour discrimination based on a non-parvocellular pathway. *Current Biology* **6**, 200–210 (1996).

[82] Chainay, H. and Humphreys, G. W. The real-object advantage in agnosia: evidence for a role of surface and depth information in object recognition. *Cognitive Neuropsychology* **18**, 175–191 (2001).

[83] Blakemore, C. and Julesz, B. Stereoscopic depth aftereffect produced without monocular cues. *Science* **171**, 286–288 (1971).

[84] Milner, A. D. and Goodale, M. A. *The Visual Brain in Action* (Oxford: Oxford University Press, 1995).

[85] Tucker, M. and Ellis, R. On the relations between seen objects and components of potential actions. *Journal of Experimental Psychology: Human Perception and Performance* **24**, 830–846 (1998).

[86] Gibson, J. J. *The Ecological Approach to Visual Perception* (Boston: Houghton Mifflin, 1979).

[87] Humphreys, G. W. and Riddoch, M. J. *To See But Not To See: A Case of Visual Agnosia* (Hillsdale, NJ: Lawrence Erlbaum, 1987).

[88] Riddoch, M. J., Humphrey, G. W., Hardy, E., Blott, W. and Smith, A. Visual and spatial short-term memory in visual agnosia. *Cognitive Neuropsychology* **20**, 641–671 (2003).

[89] Stroop, J. R. Studies of interference in serial verbal reactions. *Journal of Experimental Psychology* **18**, 643–662 (1935).

[90] Dejerine, J. Contribution à l'étude anatomo-pathologique et clinique des différentes variétés de cécité verbale. *Mémoires de la Société de Biologie* **4**, 61–90 (1892).

[91] Howard, D. Letter-by-letter readers: evidence for parallel processing. In *Basic Processes in Reading: Visual Word Recognition* (eds D. Besner and G. W. Humphreys) (Hillsdale, NJ: Lawrence Erlbaum, 1991).

[92] Shallice, T. and Warrington, E. K. The possible role of selective attention in acquired dyslexia. *Neuropsychologia* **15**, 31–41 (1977).

[93] Osswald, K., Humphreys, G. W., and Olson, A. Words are more than the sum of their parts: evidence for detrimental effects of word-level information in alexia. *Cognitive Neuropsychology* **19**, 675–695 (2002).

[94] Farah, M. J. *Visual Agnosia* (Cambridge, MA: MIT Press, 1990).

[95] Farah, M. J. *Visual Agnosia*. 2nd edn (Cambridge, MA: MIT Press, 2004).

[96] Buxbaum, L. J., Grosser, G. and Coslett, H. B. Impaired face and word recognition with object agnosia. *Neuropsychologia* **37**, 41–50 (1999).

[97] Rumiati, R. I., Humphreys, G. W., Riddoch, M. J. and Bateman, A. Visual object agnosia without prosopagnosia or alexia: evidence for hierarchical theories of object recognition. *Visual Cognition* **1**, 181–225 (1994).

[98] Rumiati, R. I. and Humphreys, G. W. Visual object agnosia without alexia or prosopagnosia: arguments for separate processing mechanisms. *Visual Cognition* **4**, 207–218 (1997).

[99] Riddoch, M. J., Humphreys, G. W., Gannon, T., Blott, W. and Jones, V. Memories are made of this: the effects of time on stored visual knowledge in a case of visual agnosia. *Brain* **122**, 537–559 (1999).

[100] Thomas, R. M., Forde, E. M. E., Humphreys, G. W. and Graham, K. S. The effects of the passage of time on a patient with category-specific agnosia. *Neurocase* **8**, 466–479 (2002).
[101] Humphreys, G. W. and Riddoch, M. J. in *Cognitive Neuropsychology and Cognitive Rehabilitation* (eds M. J. Riddoch and G. W. Humphreys) (Hillsdale, NJ: Lawrence Erlbaum, 1994).

Index

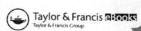
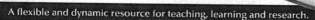